SPORTING INJURIES

Peter Dornan is a physiotherapist with more than twenty years' practical experience in the field of sporting injuries. He has been official physiotherapist for many international sporting teams, and was a foundation member of the National Rugby League Coaching Panel. A sportsman himself, he is a fellow of the Australian Sports Medicine Federation and was inaugural secretary of the Queensland branch. He has travelled extensively in the interests of sports medicine, and has written numerous articles for physiotherapy and sports medicine journals, as well as designing and marketing a video exercise program.

Richard Dunn became keenly interested in sport and sports injury rehabilitation on his return from Vietnam, where he fought as a national serviceman. In 1980 he was awarded a degree in physiotherapy from the University of Queensland. He has been official physiotherapist for many rugby and soccer teams, and toured New Zealand and France/Italy with the Wallabies. He is now working with Peter Dornan, and has written several journal articles on sports medicine. He also lectures in sports medicine for the Queensland branch of the Australian Sports Medicine Federation.

SPORTING INJURIES

Indispensable for players, coaches, teachers, parents, and all fitness enthusiasts

Peter Dornan
Richard Dunn

Drawings by Peter Dornan

University of Queensland Press
ST LUCIA • LONDON • NEW YORK

To Ronda and Hugh

P.D.

To Debra

R.D.

First published 1987 by University of Queensland Press
Box 42, St Lucia, Queensland, Australia

© Peter Dornan and Richard Dunn 1987

Typeset by Midland Typesetters, Maryborough
Printed in Australia by The Book Printer

Distributed in the UK and Europe by University of Queensland Press
Dunhams Lane, Letchworth, Herts. SG6 1LF England

Distributed in the USA and Canada by University of Queensland Press
250 Commercial Street, Manchester, NH 03101 USA

Cataloguing in Publication Data

National Library of Australia

Dornan, Peter, 1943— .
   Sporting injuries.

   Bibliography.
   Includes index.

   1. Sports — Accidents and injuries — Treatment.   2. Sports medicine.
I. Dunn, Richard. II. Title.

617'.1027

British Library (data available)

Library of Congress

Dornan, Peter, 1943— .
   Sporting injuries.

Includes bibliographies and index.
   1. Sports—Accidents and injuries. 2. Wounds and injuries — Patients —
Rehabilitation. I. Title. II. Dunn, Richard. [DNLM: 1. Athletic Injuries —
rehabilitation — handbooks. 2. Sports Medicine — methods — handbooks.
QT 39 D693s]

| RD97.D67 | 1988 | 617'.1027 | 87-5960 |

ISBN 0 7022 2064—7

CONTENTS

ACKNOWLEDGMENTS

We are indebted to the following people who have helped with various sections in certain specialist areas: Prof. Margaret Bullock (Wound Healing), Dr Tony Parker (Functional Anatomy), and Dr Brian Quigley (Exercise Physiology). We would also like to thank Mrs Roslyn Berta who patiently and skilfully deciphered, decoded, and typed our manuscript.

GLOSSARY OF TERMS

Abduction   A movement of a part away from the body
Adduction   A movement of a part towards the body
Analgesia   A decrease in the sensation of pain without loss of consciousness
Analgesic   A drug that produces analgesia
Anoxia   A lack of oxygen
Anterior   Situated towards the front or central
Anteversion   A tilting or displacement forward of a body part
Articulation   The process of being united by a joint or joints
Atrophy   A reduction in size of a muscle or region of the body
Bursa   A small sac filled with synovial fluid that allows muscle or tendon to slide over bone
Chondromalacia   Softening and destruction of the cartilage covering the articular surfaces of bones
Contra lateral   On the opposite side of the body
Crepitus   A grating sound or feeling sometimes found in fractures, tendonitis and joint pathologies
Dislocation   The displacement of one or more bones of a joint totally out of the natural joint positions
Distal   Furthest away from the centre or midline of the body
Dorsiflexion   Bending the foot towards the upper surface of the foot
Ecchymosis   Bleeding visible beneath skin causing a blue or purple discolouration
Eversion   A turning outwards
Extension   A straightening out of a flexed joint
External Rotation   Rotation of a body part towards the midline
Fascia   The fibrous tissue lying between muscles, forming the sheaths around muscles and other structures such as nerves and blood vessels
Flexion   The bending of a joint
Haemarthrosis   Blood within a joint
Haematoma   A collection of blood usually clotted which forms a mass within the tissues following trauma to the blood vessels

Haemorrhage   An escape of blood from blood vessels through damaged walls

Hypertrophy   An increase in size of a body part

Hypothermia   A reduction of body temperature to below normal which slows physiologic processes

Hypoxia   A state of oxygen want or deficiency of tissues

Inflammation   The reaction of tissues to injury characterized by heat, swelling, redness and pain

Internal Rotation   Rotation of a body part towards the midline

Inversion   A turning inwards

Lateral   Away from the midline of the body

Ligament   A band of flexible tough fibrous tissue which connects bone to bone of joints

Manipulation   1. The skilful use of hands to move joints and muscles

2. A treatment technique used to obtain forced passive movement of a joint

Medial   Towards the midline of the body

Microtrauma   Minor insignificant injury which if occurring repeatedly will give rise to an obvious injury

Neuromuscular   Pertaining to both nerves and muscles

Oedema   Excessive accumulation of fluid in tissues and joints

Osteoarthritis   A degenerative disease affecting joints

Plantar Flexion   Bending the foot downwards towards the sole

Podiatrist   A health professional who deals with the study and treatment of the feet

Posterior   Situated towards the rear or dorsal

Pronation   The turning of the palm of the hand downwards and the lowering of the arch of the foot

Proprioception   Part of the nervous system which provides the appreciation of balance, equilibrium and changes in muscle length and joint position

Proximal   Near to the body or midline of the body

Refractory   Resisting normal treatment measures

Rehabilitation   The restoration of function to damaged areas of the body

Sprain   An injury to a ligament

Strain   An injury involving the muscle, tendon or musculo-tendinous unit

Subluxation   Incomplete or partial dislocation of a joint

Supination   The turning of the palm of the hand upwards and the raising of the arch of the foot

Synovium   A membrane lining the joint capsule, bursa and tendon sheaths and producing the *synovial fluid* found in these structures

Tendon   A band of fibrous tissue attaching muscle to bone

Trauma   An injury to tissue caused by a mechanical or physical agent

Unilateral   On the same side of the body

Valgus   An abnormal turning away from the midline of the body, or as in Genu Valgum (knocked knees), an abnormal turning inwards

Varus   An abnormal turning inwards towards the midline of the body, or as in Genu Varum (bow leg), an abnormal turning outwards

Vascular   Pertaining to the blood vessels

INTRODUCTION

This book grew from the authors' need for a vehicle to instruct their patients further on the management of their soft tissue injuries. If patients fully understand the mechanisms of their injury, the pathology of wound healing and repair, plus the appropriate rehabilitative steps they must take to achieve effective healing, the possibility of a full recovery is enhanced.

Sporting Injuries discusses the current scientific knowledge of soft tissue injury management, backed and reinforced by our own clinical experience. The book is written in a non-academic style easily read by a layperson. However, we feel it may also have value for the general medical practitioner or physiotherapist who doesn't have a special interest in sports injuries, but from time to time may be consulted by a patient with a soft tissue sporting injury.

This book has evolved from Peter Dornan's first book, *Sporting Injuries: A Trainer's Guide*, which has proven to be an extremely popular publication and is used extensively as an educational guide. It was written "to assist the trainer of a sports team in the management of any injuries that may occur." The "trainer" was a term used to describe a coach, manager, fellow player or an interested onlooker who assumed responsibility for assisting an injured athlete.

Since the publication of that first book, there has been a tremendous increase in the popularity of sport and recreational pursuits such as running, cycling, swimming, aerobics, marathons, triathlons, bush walking and so on, as opposed to the traditional team sports. Consequently there has been an explosion of the newest challenge in sports medicine — the "overuse" injury.

Coupled with this increased participation and intensity in sport, there have been many recent advances in clinical and applied research in the sports sciences and in sports medicine. This book, therefore, is also intended to update and expand some of those areas related to soft tissue injury management.

The word "trainer" has been deleted in this book, as the term has evolved in different countries to mean many things, and it is not our aim to define what a trainer is or what his or her responsibilities are.

Further, the new book is not intended to be a definitive text on sports medicine or a concise first aid manual. Because of our professional training as physiotherapists, and our clinical experience with soft tissue sports injuries, we have confined the book to topics related to soft tissue injuries and their management.

Full descriptions of other topics in sports medicine, such as medical treatments, diet and nutrition, exercise physiology, biomechanics and drugs in sport have been left to the appropriate texts.

The book is divided into four parts. Part I studies "The Prevention and Nature of Injury". The leading chapter of the book is on injury prevention, as we believe that prevention is better than cure. The second chapter in part I deals with the body's response to injury via the healing processes, to establish a rationale for the use of exercise as the primary rehabilitation tool.

Part II of the book presents the principles of the management of injuries. Topics covered include the immediate management of the injured player, and a discussion of the concepts and principles of rehabilitation.

Parts III and IV of the book discuss a wide variety of soft tissue injuries. Part III has chapters covering traumatic injuries to the various joints and muscles plus neck and back pain in sport. Part IV covers the topics of overuse injuries and musculoskeletal problems peculiar to the child athlete.

In summary, we have attempted to present an informative guide to soft tissue sports injuries, providing practical suggestions for early management and principles of rehabilitation. The book is intended to help educate the injured athlete or the interested layperson, as well as to serve as a handy reference for the health professional. Obviously, we have left out precise descriptions of certain procedures, in particular, the mobilising and manipulation techniques, as we feel they are the province of the trained health professional. However, we have discussed in depth most treatment modalities and provided a rationale for their use.

PART I
THE PREVENTION
AND NATURE OF
INJURY

1
THE PREVENTION OF INJURY IN SPORT

Athletic performance today draws nearer and nearer to physiological limits and maximal human performance. Therefore, a fine line exists between injury-free performance and the overstressing of the human body. Injury is the result of stress placed upon an organism which disrupts its structure and function and results in the pathological process of repair.

CLASSIFICATION OF INJURY

Injuries can involve many factors. It is necessary to consider details such as the physical fitness of the athlete, proficiency, psychological state and nutritional state. To gain a clear appreciation of the manner in which injury develops and to illustrate the complexity of sports injury, a classification of sports injury by causative factors (adapted from Williams 1980) is presented in table 1.1.

There will always be injuries when people are involved in sport and recreation. Steps can be taken, however, to reduce the frequency and minimise the severity of injury. In industry it has been demonstrated that the prevention of injury at the worksite is far more cost effective than treating the injury after it occurs. Obviously, the same applies to the sports arena. Surgery, hospitalisation and time off work for healing and rehabilitation place enormous financial burdens on the community.

There are many factors, as illustrated in table 1.1, which can contribute to the development of an injury. The athlete has direct control over many of these factors. Athletes should ensure that they have adequate fitness levels for sport, utilise effective warm-up and warm-down procedures, use the appropriate clothing and protective devices and not infringe laws of the game to place themselves, or other participants, in danger. Other factors are not under the control of the athletes but are within the province of sports coaches, administrators and umpires. Such areas include

Table 1.1   A classification of injury in sport.

Consequential injury (due to sports participation)
PRIMARY
Extrinsic
1. Human — body contact sports (e.g. footballers' ''corked thigh'' caused by an opponent's knee).
2. Implemental — caused by racquets, bats, balls and implements necessary to carry out games.
   (a) Instantaneous — due to immediate direct violence (e.g. blow received from a hockey stick).
   (b) Overuse — repeated stress of manipulating a sporting appliance (e.g. blisters on a rower's hand).
3. Vehicular (e.g. motor cycle rider's crash).
4. Environmental — situations such as poor playing surface, bad lighting, faulty or damaged implements, extreme weather conditions.

Intrinsic (stress developed within the body)
1. Instantaneous — a sprinter's pulled hamstring.
2. Overuse.
   (a) Acute — occurring in one incidence of sports participation (e.g. Achilles tendon strain).
   (b) Chronic — developing over a period (e.g. Achilles tendonitis).

SECONDARY
This injury occurs as a result of earlier injury which has been poorly treated or poorly diagnosed.
Early
Developing soon after the primary injury (e.g. quadriceps extensor mechanism malfunction).
Late
Developing years after the injury (e.g. degenerative joint disease in an unstable knee joint).

Non-consequential injury
Injury and other conditions not directly caused by sport but which may interfere with sports participation.

Source: J.G.P. Williams, *Injury in sport,* Wolfe Medical Productions (1980).

the imparting of the specific skills and techniques of sports, providing and maintaining correct, safe, hygienic facilities for sport, and ensuring the sport is played according to the appropriate rules and in the right spirit of friendly competition.

PREVENTATIVE MEASURES

The preventative measures for minimising injury in sport have been grouped by the authors into six headings:
- pre-season medical examination;
- fitness and training;

- the warm-up;
- athletic skill and coaching proficiency;
- protective equipment;
- miscellaneous factors. They are discussed below.

PRE-SEASON MEDICAL EXAMINATION

A thorough medical examination should be undertaken and recorded at the beginning of every season. The purpose of the examination is to:
- determine if there is any defect or condition which might place the athlete at risk or increase the chance of injury and;
- bring to the attention of the coach/athlete any weaknesses or imbalances, so that these problems can be corrected.

FITNESS AND TRAINING

Inadequate fitness or conditioning is a major factor contributing to sporting injuries. A lack of strength, power, endurance, flexibility or co-ordination at a vital moment may easily lead to the breakdown of the body's tissues. The determined athlete's will to win will soon reveal a weak link resulting from a poorly designed training program.

The acquisition of fitness is a process of progressively adapting the body throughout training to withstand the rigours of competition. The purpose of training is to expose the body to repeated stresses of varying intensities and durations so that the body will adapt to these stresses. Training science determines the demands on the athlete so that improvements will occur, and the stress will not become so severe as to prevent the body from being able to adapt, with eventual injury occurring. This book does not give a complete discourse on training technique; however, there are certain principles it is necessary to grasp.

Principles of Training

- progressive overload;
- specificity;
- relaxation;
- routine.

Progressive Overload

The training program must be increased progressively so that the body is gradually challenged and placed under additional stress. Careful planning is needed, as steadily augmented practice sessions should eliminate calf and shin soreness and most of the minor muscle strains associated with overtraining. A progressive overload is implemented by increasing one or more of the following components:

- the amount of resistance;
- the repetition of sets;
- the intensity (rate) of the exercise;
- the duration of the work or exercise;

Specificity

Specificity is the overriding consideration in the planning and implementation of all training programs. The type of program must apply the appropriate stress to the specific components of the athlete's body to enable him or her to undertake a specific task. Therefore one must consider the type of sport and the position in the team for which the individual is training.
Examples:
Rugby   As well as a general conditioning program, the outside backs should concentrate on strengthening their calves, quadriceps and hamstrings; the front row forwards should concentrate on strengthening their backs, shoulder and neck muscles for scrummaging.
Running   The design of a program for 100-metre sprinters would be vastly different to that set for a marathon runner.

Relaxation

The body needs time to recover from hard exercise routines. Adequate rest is necessary to allow recuperation and repair of any damage suffered during a hard training session. Training should allow for "hard-easy" days. Heavy sessions should occur only three to four times a week with light workouts in between. A lack of adequate rest or sleep may result in either physiological staleness, characterised by a decreased ability to perform and muscle fatigue, or psychological staleness, characterised by a loss of interest in training or competing.

Routine

Fitness training is a continual process and it must be done regularly, year in year out. As well as an overall season plan, there should be both a weekly and a daily plan. It is the responsibility of the coach to monitor the athletes' performance, making sure they are not overworked, that they are getting adequate sleep and that they are on a proper diet.

Components of Fitness

Physical fitness can be broken down into a number of components, namely:
1   Cardiovascular endurance;
2   Muscular strength, power and endurance; and
3   Flexibility.
It is important to understand how each of these components adapts to the rigours of training.

1   Cardiovascular Endurance

The ability of the athlete to sustain repeated muscular effort requires the respiratory system, the heart and the blood vessels to deliver fuel and oxygen to muscles at a rate fast enough to prolong the time before fatigue sets in. Fatigue will leave the athlete vulnerable to injury.

"Aerobic training" is the term used to describe the development of cardiovascular endurance, and certain variables must be considered to gain the necessary adaptations:

Intensity of the program   Setting the intensity of a program can be easily determined by the response of the heart rate to exercise. The maximum heart rate of an individual can be calculated by a simple formula: 220 minus the age of the individual. Therefore the maximum heart rate for a twenty-year-old would be around 200 beats per minute. To gain an increase in cardiovascular endurance an athlete should work at 80 per cent of his or her maximal heart rate; in the case of the twenty-year-old, this would be 160 beats per minute. It is important to remember that as cardiovascular endurance improves, the heart rate will drop.

Duration of workout   A workout session of at least 30 minutes maintaining the target heart rate is the minimum necessary to produce significant adaptation.

Frequency of workout   The minimum number is three sessions of aerobic activity per week.

The cardiovascular system will adapt to exercise in various ways:

- the heart, which is a specialised muscle, will develop in thickness and therefore become a more efficient pump producing an increased stroke volume and cardiac output, increasing blood supply to the muscles;
- there will be an increased ability to extract oxygen from the air breathed into the lungs;
- the blood vessels, especially the smaller ones (capillaries), will show a decrease in resistance to blood flow.

Anaerobic conditioning   The anaerobic system is the local muscle energy system that is used in the absence of oxygen. It is used in explosive body movements which occur before oxygen can be delivered to the muscle. To train this system, rapid explosive movements of short duration are necessary, for example, short distance sprints. Therefore, a training program should strike a balance between long distance endurance work (aerobic) and short, intensive fast speed work (anaerobic).

2   Muscular Parameters

A muscle can develop increases in strength, power and endurance.
Strength   This is defined as the maximum force developed by a muscle against a resistance, and is proportional to the cross-sectional area of the muscle. When a muscle is subjected to high intensity demands, it will respond by increasing in size and strength. Best strength gains are achieved by a high resistance-low repetition regime. Steps in determining a strength program are to select:

- the type of resistance (table 1.2);
- the amount of weight or resistance to be applied;
- the number of repetitions per set;
- the number of sets per workout;
- the number of workouts per week.

Power   This is the rate of doing work. It is the ability of the muscle to exert a force at accelerated speed, therefore explosive contractions are required. The best apparatuses available to develop power are the isokinetic devices.
Endurance   This is the ability of the muscle to contract repeatedly. Athletes not only need to develop appropriate levels of strength, but they also need to use a high percentage of that strength over a period of time through repeated muscular

Table 1.2   Types of resistance used in strength training.

Types of resistance	Type of movement	Device used
Isometric	No movement, contraction against a fixed resistance; each contraction held for six seconds	Any immovable object
Isotonic	These are contractions where the muscle changes length against a resistance	Free weights Wall pulleys e.g. Universal, Nautilus
Isokinetic	These contractions require a specialized device which allows an accommodating resistance; that is, the resistance adapts throughout the range of motion	Cybex, Orthotron, Hydragym

contractions. Best endurance gains are achieved with moderate resistance-high repetitions. To set an endurance program:

- select a low resistance;
- increase the rate of work;
- increase the number of repetitions and sets.

3   Flexibility

A lack of flexibility is a common cause of injury to muscles and joints. Increasing flexibility through stretching may decrease the incidence of musculotendinous injury, minimise and alleviate muscle soreness, and contribute to improved athletic performance. It has been demonstrated that it is necessary for a muscle to achieve full stretch before it can attain full power. Similarly, a ligament or tendon must have sufficient length to allow a joint to move fully through its normal range of motion and achieve efficient function. Therefore, to prevent injury, athletes should carry out regular stretching exercises to ensure the flexibility and range of motion of joints and muscles.

The stretching technique and the methods used to incorporate stretching exercises in an overall fitness plan are crucial to the development of a safe, effective program. Poor technique and improper stretching may actually cause musculotendinous injury. Increases in flexibility should be attained by slow gentle *static* stretches. Static stretching allows the muscle's protective reflex, the stretch reflex, to be overcome. The muscle is then relaxed and can be stretched further safely. The athlete should hold the position of stretch for 10 to 15 seconds. There should be *NO* excess straining, bouncing or pain. As flexibility improves, the duration of the stretch can be increased to 30 or more seconds. This is the safest and most effective method of gaining increases in flexibility.

Ballistic stretches (for example, high kicks), "bouncing" in the stretched position, or rapid movements during a stretch are all counterproductive. The reason is that a muscle will reflexively contract when it is suddenly stretched (the stretch reflex). Therefore, any fast bouncing stretch will be against a contracted muscle which may injure the muscle tissue if it is forced, or will not produce any significant stretching of the muscle. Slow, static stretching on the other hand will override the stretch reflex and allow the muscle to increase in length.

Planning a Stretching Program   It is important to realise that increasing flexibility is a gradual progression and it will take many weeks for any benefit to occur. Athletes should be encouraged to develop a year-round program. Stretching at the beginning of a season will only have minimal benefits.

Stretching should always be preceded by a mild "aerobic" warm-up; that is, a mild, repetitive activity such as jogging or cycling (see the "Warm-up" section later in this chapter). The reason is that warming muscles increases their extensibility which helps protect the muscles against injury and allows for greater gains in flexibility.

Stretching and an effective warm-up should precede all physical activity. Further stretching can also be undertaken during a workout routine when the muscles are warm and extensible. Stretching after a heavy workout is an excellent way to relax muscles and minimise muscle soreness.

Muscle groups should be alternated throughout the stretching routine. If, for example, the routine starts with a quadriceps stretch, the next exercise should be for some other group, such as the calf muscles. Spacing of various exercises will avoid the exertion of excessive force on a muscle group.

Stretching Summary

- Precede stretching with a mild "aerobic" warm-up.
- Use the static stretching technique.
- The stretching position should be assumed slowly and gently until tightness is experienced. This position is held for 15 or more seconds. There should be *no pain, no bouncing or jerky movements*.
- Exercise the various muscle groups alternately.
- Stretch before, after and if possible during exercise sessions.

If there is time for only one routine, stretching before activity is the most important.

• Plan a year-round stretching routine.

Basic stretches for the important muscle groups are shown in figures 1.1 to 1.3.

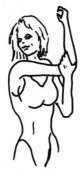

a. Shoulders.

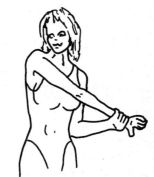

Pull one elbow across to the opposite shoulder.

Pull one arm across the body, thumb towards the ground.

b. Biceps.

c. Triceps.

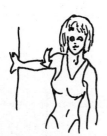

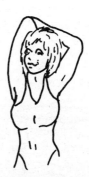

Hold onto a door at arms' length, thumb down. Turn the body away from that arm; let the shoulder roll in.

Place one hand behind the head. Pull the elbow behind the head with the opposite hand.

Figure 1.1 Stretches for the upper limbs.

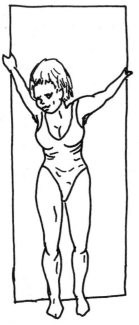

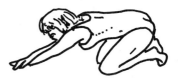

e. Latissimus dorsi.

Raise the hands over the head, and stretch forward as shown. Then, with hips in the air and hands on the floor, lean hips towards the side to be stretched. Feel the stretch from the shoulderblade to armpit.

d. Pectoral muscles.

Stand in a doorway. Lean the body forwards.

g. Wrist/forearm extensors.

With elbow straight, pull on the back of the hand.

f. Wrist/forearm flexors.

With a straight elbow, pull on the palm of the hand till the stretch is felt in the forearm.

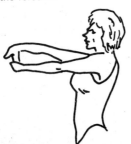

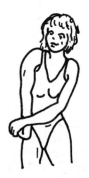

Figure 1.1 Stretches for the upper limbs (continued).

a. Back extensors.

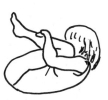

Curl into a ball.

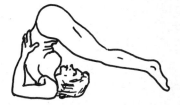

Bring the legs over the head — use the hands to keep balance.

c. Side flexors.

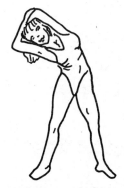

b. Abdominals.

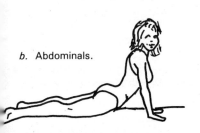

Rest the hips on the floor; stretch up with the trunk.

Stand with the feet apart, hands grasping the opposite elbows above the head. Bend to one side, taking elbows towards the hip.

Figure 1.2 Stretches for the trunk.

Partner stretching—the contract relax method Many athletes find that they have some muscle groups that are particularly tight and find difficulty in relaxing them to gain significant stretching. Partner stretching is an effective tool to aid these athletes. The basic procedure is this:

(a) The athlete moves the limb in the direction to be stretched until a feeling of tension is experienced. This position is held for ten seconds.

(b) The limb is then forced against a resistance applied by the

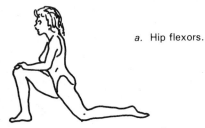

a. Hip flexors.

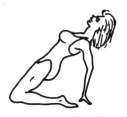

Kneel as shown, and lean forward, keeping the pelvis forward and the back straight.

Lean back until the stretch is felt at the top of the thigh.

b. Quadriceps.

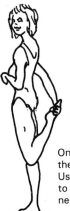

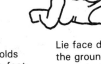

One hand holds the opposite foot. Use the other hand to balance if necessary.

Lie face down. Keeping the pelvis on the ground, stretch one thigh off the ground with the opposite arm.

c. Adductors.

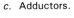

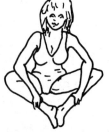

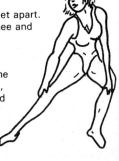

Push the knees towards the floor.

Stand up, feet apart. Bend one knee and shift body weight to that side, stretching the opposite leg, which is held straight.

Figure 1.3   Stretches for the lower limbs.

d. Hamstrings.

Lie on your back. Pull one thigh up
with both hands, then straighten
the knee.

Standing up,
place one leg
on a bench.
Bend the
opposite knee
to lock low
back. With
back straight,
lean forwards.

Turn each foot in to stretch the
lateral hamstrings — out to stretch
the medial hamstrings.

f. Buttock stretch.

e. Outer thigh.

Place the leg to
be stretched
behind the
other leg,
keeping the
first leg
straight. Let the
front knee relax
as you rotate
and bend away
from the leg to
be stretched.

Keep both
buttocks on the
ground, with
the back
straight. Press
against one
knee as shown,
while turning
that leg away
from the body.

Figure 1.3 Stretches for the lower limbs (continued).

g. Calf muscles.

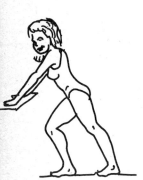 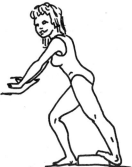 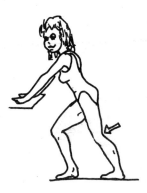

To stretch the gastrocnemius muscle, have the feet and body pointing forward, back straight. Lean forward; the heels must remain on the ground.

A better stretch can be obtained by using an incline board.

To stretch the soleus muscle, use the same position as for the gastrocnemius, then bend the knee to isolate the soleus.

Figure 1.3   Stretches for the lower limbs (continued).

partner in the *opposite* direction to that being stretched. The partner provides an isometric resistance (no movement) and the contraction is held for six seconds.

(c) Following relaxation of the muscle, it is moved by the partner gently in the direction to be stretched and again held for ten seconds at the new position of stretch.

The procedure is repeated four or five times and relaxation of the muscle and an increase in flexibility will be noted if it is done correctly. Precise descriptions of these techniques are not presented as they can only be taught by someone experienced in their use.

THE WARM-UP

The warm-up is an integral part of injury prevention as it prepares the athlete's body and mind for competition. A warm-up should be designed to fulfil five main requirements. It should:

- ensure complete flexibility of all joints and muscles;
- ensure proper muscle contractility for sudden explosive action;

Table 1.3 Summary of training components and their role in injury prevention.

Training components	Definition	Application to injury prevention
Cardiovascular endurance	The ability of the lungs, heart and vascular system to deliver fuel and oxygen to the muscles	To ensure a continuous supply of oxygen and fuel to muscles; to avoid the onset of fatigue
Strength	Maximum force developed by a muscle	To stabilise an anatomical area against applied forces
Power	Rate of doing work	To ensure muscles can respond quickly to the threat of injury
Endurance	Ability of the muscle to repeatedly contract	To avoid low endurance levels, which lead to early fatigue and hence injury
Flexibility	The range of motion a joint is permitted by the muscles and surrounding tissues	To respond to forced extensibility without injury
Skill	Balance, co-ordination, agility	To control body movements

- raise aerobic energy supply;
- refresh skill patterns;
- aid psychological preparation for sport.

Exercise increases body temperatures and flexibility increases as body temperature rises. It has been found that an increase in muscle temperature enables enzyme systems to work more rapidly and improves the viscosity of tissues. This increases the speed at which the muscle is able to contract and attain optimal performance. The athlete's body tends to work more efficiently and safely when a thorough warm-up has elevated core temperature.

The essential fuel, oxygen, must be transported from the outside air via the cardiovascular system (aerobic energy) to supplement the immediate source of energy contained in the muscles (anaerobic energy). A slow, steady run will raise the maximum oxygen uptake, elevate the heart rate and reduce the resistance to blood flow, therefore attaining the maximum efficiency of the aerobic energy supply system. If fast powerful sprinting work is done too early the athlete will use up anaerobic energy supply before the aerobic supply can reach the muscle, causing the lactate level (waste products) in the blood to rise and this will lead to early fatigue.

Where possible, the warm-up session should reproduce the actual movements of the sport to be played. This will activate the neuromuscular pathways which are necessary to attain the specific skills of a sport, such as passing, throwing, kicking and so on.

Warm-up sessions should also be used for the psychological preparation necessary for competition. A clever coach will use this period as a positive cue in the "psyching" procedure necessary for top performance. The days of the old "yelling and abuse" style of "psyche up" are gone. A slow controlled approach is now favoured where the mind is tuned into the job to be done by the visualisation of the event and the practice of specific skills that the athlete will be required to perform.

The intensity and duration of a warm-up should be governed by the type of event and the fitness of the athlete. As a general rule, trained athletes should warm up for approximately twenty to thirty minutes before competing. It is important for the athlete to be aware of the need to stay warm until competition starts and remain warm during the actual event, for instance, a rugby winger waiting for the ball to come his way must continually stretch and exercise to stay warm if he wants to avoid muscle or joint injury.

A Typical Warm-Up Routine

1 Slow steady jog for approximately five minutes. Slow jogging will raise the aerobic capacity and increase core temperature of the body.
2 Stretching routine — approximately ten minutes. This routine should stretch all major joints and muscles starting at the neck and systematically working down the body. Special attention must be placed on the muscles of the lower limbs and back which are more susceptible to injury.
3 Running — approximately five minutes. Progressive running drills over varying distances and increasing speeds should be given until the athlete has reached full pace over 75 to 100 metres. Leg stretches should be interspersed with running drills.
4 Skill — approximately ten minutes. The activities and skills that the athlete will perform during the event should be practised during this period. For example, netball players should practise passing and goal shooting; sprinters their starts; and footballers kicking and passing plus running through the planned "moves" that the team sports will attempt during the course of the match.
5 Rest. A period of ten minutes or so should be allowed for the athlete to relax before competition. Last-minute equipment and

clothing checks should be carried out and the final psychological preparations completed.

6 Warm-down. After the event a three- to five-minute warm-down should be allowed. This removes waste products (lactates) from the muscles and may be helpful in reducing much of the post-match stiffness and soreness. Stretching of tired muscles will also aid in their relaxation.

ATHLETIC SKILL AND COACHING PROFICIENCY

The role of the coach in imparting the correct techniques and skills of the sport to the athletes is an important factor in maintaining injury-free performance. For example, an incorrect technique in a javelin throw can lead to elbow injury; the fast bowler with an improper action may suffer low back pain; and an excessive "whip kick" may cause pain to develop in the breaststroker's knee. In many sports coaches are appointed on the basis of their former prowess. These coaches are always well intentioned but often lack scientific knowledge concerning fitness training, skill development and injury prevention. Most sports now run courses that coaches must do to gain "accreditation" and enable them to be considered as coaches to senior teams and elite competitors. However, many children are still exposed to unqualified coaches with some disastrous results.

Referees and coaches also have a responsibility to ensure that athletic endeavour is carried out within the rules and spirit of the game. Acts of premeditated violence, or intentional cheating risking injury to an opponent, are abhorrent. One of the most emotive issues in sports injury is the prevalence of catastrophic spinal injuries in the football codes. Many of these injuries are unavoidable accidents, while others are due to acts of violence such as "spear tackles". Scrums account for the majority of these injuries and the causative factors are basically twofold: poor scrummaging skill/technique; and cheating, through incorrect binding such as loose arms or intentional collapsing to gain advantage.

The elimination of these disastrous injuries lies well within the areas of responsibility of sports administration, coaches and referees.

PROTECTIVE EQUIPMENT

The prime example of the use of protective devices in sport is the equipment used in American gridiron football. No other sport has such a vast array of body protective pads, guards, facial protectors and strapping as American football. Cricket is also becoming a gladiatorial game, due to the strength and power of the modern fast bowler. Consequently, in the last few years there has been an increasing growth in the variety of protective equipment used by batters to protect vulnerable parts of their bodies from damage caused by the impact of the cricket ball. Figure 1.4 depicts the type of padding now commonly available to cricketers.

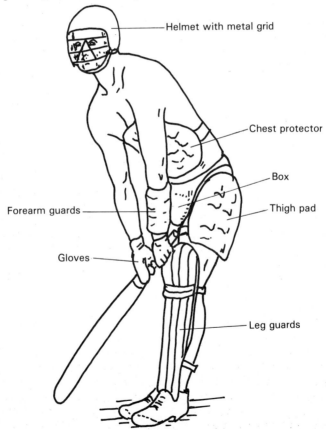

Figure 1.4 Cricket protection equipment needed to face a modern fast bowler.

Protective equipment used in sport must incorporate the following features in its design:

- Construction should be of light materials, comfortable to wear and allowing adequate ventilation, particularly in a hot climate.
- The device should not restrict movement or the normal function of the body. Protective equipment should not hinder the athlete's ability to perform.
- The design of a protective device should be appropriate for the sport being played, and not breach the rules of the sport or be used as a weapon. In many sports there are no design specifications for protective equipment;, therefore, poorly designed or inappropriate devices can give a false sense of security.
- A protective device should be constructed of materials capable of reducing the full force of impact over the body part to be protected.

Helmets

Helmets must be worn in activities where the head and face are at risk of injury by forceful contact. Sports where helmets are worn include: American football, motor racing, cycling, BMX riding, horse riding, cricket and ice hockey. Each sport has different design requirements, therefore a helmet designed for horse riding would not be suitable for motor racing.

Certain sports need helmets that have attachments to protect the face and eyes, for example cricket and ice hockey. Facial protection is gained by either a steel mesh mask or a perspex visor. Helmets and their attachments must be light in construction, comfortable, able to absorb impact and not restrict vision.

It is essential to encourage children to wear safety helmets in many sports and recreational pursuits, especially activities such as cycling, BMX riding, skate boarding and cricket. Many serious head injuries and deaths can be prevented by the use of this simple readily available device.

Headgear

In days gone by, headgear was fashionable in rugby football to protect a player's ears from trauma. Since the advent of specially designed adhesive tapes to protect the ears, headgear has lost favour. Recently, a new headgear design has emerged which may help reduce concussive impact forces as well as providing ear protection.

Eye Protection

The use of protective eye glasses is essential for squash and other racquet sports. Squash is particularly dangerous, as the ball is small enough to penetrate the eye socket deeply and cause extensive damage to the eye. Squash players compete in close proximity; therefore, accidental blows from the racquets are common also.

Goggles are valuable in sports such as skiing and motor cycle riding to protect the eyes from the wind, glare, foliage, dirt or snow. Swimmers wear specialised goggles to protect their eyes from chlorine irritation and the reflected glare of the sun in outdoor pools.

Mouthguards

Mouthguards must be worn in all contact sports, particularly all codes of football and boxing. The precise fitting of mouthguards must be done by a dentist to ensure comfort, ease of breathing and allow reasonable speech. "Over the counter" devices are at best only temporary solutions. Mouthguards are designed to protect the jaws and teeth against impact and have a role to play in reducing concussion.

Protective Padding

Various types of shoulder pads are used in sports such as American football, rugby league, motor cross, skate boarding and BMX riding. Shoulder padding does *not* protect the joints and bones of the shoulder from injuries such as dislocation of the shoulder joint, fractures of the collar bone or sprains of the acromio-clavicular joint. The role of shoulder pads is to protect the soft tissues of the shoulder region from bruising.

Padding can also be worn over other areas of the body, such as the elbow, knee, chest and thigh. These devices will only protect the underlying soft tissues from blows and impact forces. The design and type of padding used must be appropriate for the sport and be within the rules of the game.

Guards

Elastic guards do not protect joints from injury or support and protect injured joints from re-injury. Their main use is in applying compression to reduce swelling in a damaged joint. In certain knee conditions, especially those involving the kneecap, types of guards available on the market are made of a material that retains body temperature and may play a role in the rehabilitative stage after injury.

The shin must be protected from impact in sports such as field hockey, soccer and certain rugby positions. Shin guards should be made of a material that will protect the sensitive areas from impact as well as fitting and moulding to the leg comfortably.

Bracing

Bracing of joints, particularly the knee, is becoming widespread in north American sport. Bracing can be divided into three distinct areas: prophylactic (preventing injury), rehabilitative and functional.

To the authors' knowledge, prophylatic knee bracing has not been attempted in Australian sport to any degree. There are few studies to support its effectiveness and its use is questionable in contact sports where braces could be used as a weapon. Various forms of light ankle braces are available and are popular in basketball and netball. At this stage it is difficult to give an informed opinion on whether ankle braces are as effective in joint protection as prophylatic ankle taping.

Bracing is an orthopaedic procedure commonly used to facilitate rehabilitation of a joint following surgery to repair joint structures. The type, design and use of the brace remain the prerogative of the orthopaedic surgeon.

Functional braces are designed to support a joint which is unstable due to extensive damage to ligaments of the joint. This type of bracing is popular overseas, particularly in the United States. However, it is difficult to assess the effectiveness of braces as there has been little research into their use. There are many designs and combinations of braces for the knee and shoulder joints. Orthopaedic consultation should be sought for the prescription of the appropriate device.

Taping

There is a reasonable body of evidence to suggest that taping of ankles in contact sport will help prevent the incidence of ankle joint injuries. Sports where ankles should be routinely taped include football, basketball, netball, hockey and volleyball. A technique of prophylatic ankle taping is described in chapter 7, and demonstrated in figure 7.47.

At present there is no evidence to support the taping of other joints of the body to prevent injury to a healthy joint. Joints and structures that are recovering from injury may derive some benefit from taping. However, taping and strapping should never replace a comprehensive rehabilitation program. If athletes cannot compete without metres of strapping to support a damaged structure the authors believe that they should not participate in sport until, through active rehabilitation, they are able to play without tape.

Clothing

Appropriate sports clothing must be selected to keep the body at a comfortable temperature. In the warm Australian climate, clothing must be designed to allow adequate ventilation to ensure heat loss through conduction, convection and evaporation of sweat. The practice of exercising with clothing to induce weight loss by sweating is strongly condemned. The weight loss occurs because of body fluid depletion and is only temporary, until body fluids are replaced. It is also a highly dangerous procedure as the cooling of the body is impeded, and, as the body's fluids deplete, serious heat stress syndrome can result.

Footwear must be appropriate for the chosen sport. In most sports shoes are the most important item in providing protection. For a detailed description of footwear, especially for runners, see chapter 9. Shock- absorbing inner soles are devices that can reduce impact shock to the legs and trunk. However, they are not a panacea for the treatment or relief of existing ailments of the limbs.

Wet suits should be worn in many aquatic sports, especially high speed activities such as water skiing and sail boarding. As well as protecting the body from the effects of inclement weather, they are extremely useful in protecting the abdominal and pelvic organs of the body, especially in females.

MISCELLANEOUS FACTORS

Diet

The appropriate food intake plays an essential role in injury prevention by supplying the necessary energy to guard against early fatigue. A well balanced nutritious diet is needed to maintain health and fitness. An excellent book on diet and sport has recently been published, *Food for Sport* (see the reading list at the end of the book).

Fluid Replenishment

An adequate intake of water is essential before and during competition and training to prevent dehydration, cramping and heart stress injury. During heavy exercise, an athlete can lose up to four to five kilograms of body fluid. Athletes should drink regularly as no matter how much people drink, they cannot keep up with fluid losses during training and competition. Consequently, athletes should ingest fluids frequently during activity and consume 400 to 500ml of fluid 10 to 15 minutes before competition and drink small amounts as often as possible during the event.

Hygiene

Athletes must be careful about their personal hygiene, for their own protection and that of their fellow athletes. This is especially important in team sports, particularly when travelling where infection and disease can easily spread to team-mates. It is essential to clean and treat all skin wounds, no matter how trivial, to prevent infection.

Sports Facilities

Care must be taken by sports administrators to provide safe sports arenas for both the athletes and the spectators. Design should take into consideration such factors as the position of the sun, providing an appropriate playing surface and avoiding the encroachment of fences and advertising hoardings. Indoor settings must have effective lighting and ventilation. All sports venues must be inspected for potential dangers before competition and have clean hygienic change rooms and toilets.

2
THE HEALING PROCESS

Sports injuries are not generally serious. Damage to tissue is usually slight and the healing capacity great. In spite of this, the healing process often takes longer than desirable. This necessity for extra time often conflicts with the patient's keenness to return to sport again at the highest level of performance possible in as short a time as possible.

Because the majority of sports injuries involve soft tissue damage (that is, ligaments, muscles, tendons, skin and so on), it is essential to understand the process of healing and repair. The fact is that wound healing at its best is imperfect. The consequent implications of this deficiency are vital for people playing sport. *In truth, appreciating and understanding this point may be the key to the successful management of soft tissue sporting injuries.*

The process of the formation of scar tissue, and its associated properties, is a particular aspect of wound healing not often satisfactorily understood.

The purpose of this chapter is to provide a rationale for the treatment of wound healing problems, based on the knowledge of the mechanisms involved in connective tissue repair together with specific clinical observations.

It will be convenient to discuss the matter under these five separate headings:
- inflammation and repair;
- factors affecting wound healing;
- healing of special tissues;
- scar tissue and patient management;
- chronic scarring syndrome.

INFLAMMATION AND REPAIR

Wound healing is a sequence in which injury is the first step, inflammation the second, fibroplasia (the growth of a fibrous tissue scar) the third, and remodelling the fourth. The most common cause of injury in sport is trauma, either from an external force or from continual repetitive stress. Other causes of injury are chemical agents (stings, acids, and so on), hot and cold extremes, radiation, bacterial and viral infections and all types of immunological reactions.

Inflammation is best defined as the local reaction of vascularised tissue to injury. It is an essential check on bacterial infections; wounds and injured tissues would never heal without the inflammatory reaction, and it is an essential step in the process of repair.

On the other hand, inflammation may be potentially harmful. With chronic inflammatory conditions or large wounds, reparative efforts often lead to disfiguring scars and fibrous bonds that limit the mobility and function of joints and organs.

The local clinical signs of inflammation are heat, redness, swelling, pain and loss of function. Immediately after injury, there is a transient vasoconstriction (tightening) of blood vessels. This is a minimal and inconsistent reaction, and is immediately followed by vasodilation (widening). This brings about increased blood flow and is the cause of the heat and redness.

The swelling is largely produced by the escape of fluid, plasma proteins and cells from the blood into the perivascular tissues, as the blood vessels lose their normal ability to retain fluids and cells. Essentially, in a localised inflammation site (for example, a strained ligament), a vascular phenomenon occurs that brings about a fluid imbalance causing white cells to concentrate at the site.

White blood cells are major contributors to the body's defence mechanisms, so their concentration at the injury site helps prevent invasion by infectious organisms.

Pain associated with injury is caused by a number of factors. First, it is produced by pressure on nerve endings as the exudative swelling increases in size. Pain can also be induced by the release of certain body chemicals, particularly histamines, at the injury site. Ischaemia (a lack of blood supply) caused by damage to the local blood vessels, will also produce pain.

The process of wound repair, called fibroplasia, consists of a chronological sequence of events which leads to the formation of a fibrous tissue scar. In soft tissue injuries two types of repair exist; healing by primary or by secondary intention.

HEALING BY FIRST INTENTION

Healing by first intention, or *primary* healing, occurs as a result of an accident or surgery which leaves a clean wound with even and closely opposed edges. Briefly, the epithelial cells of the outer surface of the cut edge migrate and proliferate rapidly to bridge the gap, as shown in figure 2.1.

Within 24 hours, large numbers of granulocytes, monocytes and lymphocytes (white blood cells) accumulate and by the end of the second day a smooth lining or endothelium has formed. By the third day small blood vessels (capillaries) sprout and by the fifth day reticular fibres are seen. These are the precursors of the collagen fibres which make up the fibrous scar. The great bulk of the collagen fibres are laid down during the second week.

At first, the scar has many blood vessels and appears red, and on cold days, blue. After some months, only a fine lamina of fibrous tissues marks the original site of the wound.

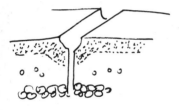

a. A clean wound — surgery or a cut.

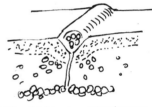

b. After 24 hours — granulocytes, monocytes and lymphocytes accumulate to form an endothelium.

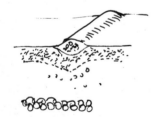

c. After 10-15 days, capillary growth is proceeding upwards from the subcutaneous tissue. Fibrosis (scarring) is far advanced. Scab falls off.

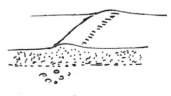

d. Months or years later — a fine lamina of fibrous tissue marks the wound site.

Figure 2.1 Healing by first intention.

HEALING BY SECOND INTENTION

Healing by second intention occurs when there is a gaping wound and the edges cannot be approximated; see figure 2.2. Immediately, fibrinogen(a protein in the blood plasma which is the precursor of a blood clot) clots on the surface covering the wound with transparent fibrin. By five to six days, the surface assumes a red and finely granular appearance. Each of the granules consists of a core of wide new capillaries, the growth of which raises the enveloping mantle of macrophages, fibroblasts and other cells into a small elevation.

The fourth stage of repair is the remodelling phase. This phase, which partially overlaps the regeneration phase, is characterised

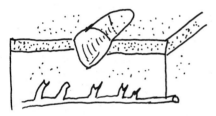

a. Immediately (within five minutes), fibrinogen clots on the surface covering the wound. The wound cavity is filled with a blood clot.

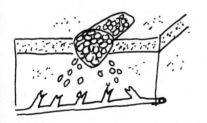

b. After six days, granulated tissue forms at the base of the wound site.

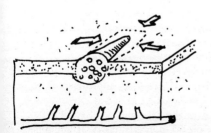

c. Three weeks after injury, macrophages and fibroblasts form fibrous granulation tissue and heal from the bottom and sides upwards to create an elevation. As the wound closes, the surrounding tissue contracts.

Figure 2.2 Healing by second intention.

by a reduction in size of the wound surface, an increase in the strength of the scar, and an alteration of the fibre structure.

As soon as regeneration of granulation tissue has occurred, *contraction takes places, a process which continues for as long as the elasticity of the surrounding fibres allows*. Current evidence suggests that wound contraction is a cellular function of contractile fibroblasts, the cells which synthesise collagen fibres.

Research has shown that in the early stages of healing, wound strength relates directly to the quality of collagen. After two or three weeks, further gains in strength are determined by the qualitative changes in these fibres. It has been suggested that the strength gain at this later stage is due to two factors: an intra-molecular and inter-molecular cross-linking of the collagen fibres, and a remodelling by dissolution and reforming of the collagen fibres, to give a stronger, more efficient weave.

The collagen is continuously turned over. Although the quantity remains constant, new fibres are formed and old ones broken down. The rate of this turnover in the first three months definitely appears to be related to the increase in strength of the scar.

This remodelling phase imposes the most important implications for the management of soft tissue injuries; that is, the rigidity and loss of extensibility plus the lack of tensile strength of scar tissue. These factors are discussed in depth in this chapter, under the section on "Scar tissue".

FACTORS AFFECTING WOUND HEALING

The final nature and quality of the wound healing product is dependent on a great number of factors.

BLOOD SUPPLY

An adequate blood supply must be present if healing is to proceed normally. Poor circulation may slow healing down. Unfortunately, the original injury often damages local circulation, so optimal conditions for tissue nutrition are achieved only if blood volume is maintained, vasoconstriction is minimised, blood supply is adequate, and fluid overloads and tissue oedema are avoided. Research has shown that the rate and quality of repair are directly proportional to the blood oxygen supply at all levels.

Heating the tissues has been found to increase the blood supply and aid the healing processes. Heating accelerates metabolism, which allows a faster exchange of nutrients and waste products. For each degree of temperature increase, the metabolic rate of the cell increases by about 13 per cent. The infrared lamp, the hot water bag, and warm showers and baths are all forms of heat that can be applied at home or in a club. In the physiotherapist's rooms, shortwave diathermy and ultrasound, which penetrate more deeply and produce as much as five to six degrees increase in temperature to a depth of 5 centimetres, are used. This increases the blood flow even more, and the heat can reach more blood vessels.

Significantly, it has also been shown that muscular work or exercise can increase the heat production ten or twenty times more than the heat production at rest.

AGE OF PATIENT

There are "natural delays" in the healing of older individuals. Researchers have found that it takes almost twice the time for complete wound closure for a 40-year-old man as it does for a 20-year-old man. Similarly, other workers in this field have found the tearing strength of wounds (scars) in older rats was significantly lower than that in younger animals. Major differences have been found in the healing patterns of young and old individuals.

Younger individuals have an earlier and greater increase in metabolism (the supply of energy) allowing for faster healing rates. Further observations suggest a similar amount of collagen but a higher rate of collagen turnover in the young. This similarity is consistent with increased modelling and implies greater strength per unit of collagen.

The effect of age on collagen is a decrease in the maximum tensile strength and a decrease in the elastic modules. The rate of adaptation to stress is slower with increasing age. The net clinical result is a marked increase in the amount of healing time plus an increase in overuse syndromes and fatigue failures in muscles and tendons in older athletes.

STEROIDS

Steroids have a deleterious effect on collagen and wound healing. Impairment of wound strength by cortisone was first reported in

1950, and has since been confirmed in numerous clinical studies. It has been found that both cortisone and methylprednisolone retard collagen accumulation in experimental granulation tissue during the first two weeks of healing. It is generally contra-indicated to inject hydro-cortisone into the lower limb weight-bearing tissues of athletes. As anyone who does not play sport regularly will generally rest after an injury, and the cortisone does have an effect of relieving pain and inflammation, non-athletes can usually tolerate steroid injections with no noticeable immediate disastrous side effects. Because of the natural weakening effect of the cortisone on the healing tissues, and other tissues, when people are tempted to overload the injured structure too soon, they will cause more damage.

IMMOBILISATION

Many negative effects on tissues become obvious after immobilisation. The rates of return of function of muscle, tendon, bone and fibrous tissue have been well studied. The effects are discussed further in this chapter under the "Scar tissue" section.

ACTIVITY AND EXERCISE

Regular cyclic loading results in increased connective tissue strength. Because of the natural weakness of healing scar tissue, there are many positive desirable effects to be gained by controlled exercise. Similarly, because of the contractile nature of scar tissue, controlled stretching exercises can re-orientate and restructure the tissues to a more functional level. This aspect of exercise is discussed more fully in this chapter under "Scar tissue".

Tension and pressure on the growing collagen fibres determine the direction in which they will lie, and if space permits, their abundance. Fibres, therefore, develop along the lines of tension. Mild tension enhances tensile strength — too much tension can be disruptive and undesirable. Repeated forceful stretching of ligament and capsular tissues will tend to increase the inflammation, resulting in more scar tissue formation, and more seriously, will continue to impair the flexibility and elasticity, further continuing the cycle. This aspect of activity is also covered more fully in this chapter, under "Scar tissue".

As mentioned earlier, exercise increases the blood supply to the injured area which can enhance the healing effect. The advantages of exercise over heat application in this context are discussed further in chapter 5, "Rehabilitation".

NERVES

Damage to sections of the nerves supplying skin, connective tissue and muscle does not alter the rate or quality of healing. Acute denervation has no effect on wound healing if the damaged point is not under stress.

SIZE OF WOUND

Epithelium, connective tissue and vessels each grow at a uniform rate throughout the period of healing. The initial size of the wound does not affect rate of growth.

OEDEMA (SWELLING)

Moderate oedema has little or no effect on tensile strenth gain. However, it has been shown that marked oedema has a slight and temporary inhibitory effect on healing. This effect may be more mechanical than biochemical in nature.

It is therefore important to keep swelling to a minimum at all stages of rehabilitation. Methods to control swelling are discussed further in chapter 3.

HEALING OF SPECIAL TISSUES

SKIN

Wound healing is a complex process involving cell movement, and people have a pattern of wound repair suited to their particular skin. Both primary and secondary types of healing have been discussed in some detail in this chapter under "Inflammation and repair".

Of clinical importance, it has been found that epithelisation is retarded by the dry scab which normally covers a superficial wound, and if the formation of a scab is prevented by keeping the wound moist (and scrupulously clean), the rate of epithelisation is markedly increased.

CARTILAGE

Cartilage possesses restricted powers of regeneration. Wounds in cartilage tissue heal by the formation of fibrous scars around which cartilage cells divide and in time replace the scar tissue. Regeneration is a slow process lasting over many weeks and apparently varies a great deal in different types of cartilage. This is particularly obvious, clinically, with rib cartilages; they may take months to heal.

Most cartilage types, though relatively non-vascular, are penetrated by numerous small canals, each conveying a small artery and vein. However, of clinical importance, articular hyaline cartilage, of which the most prominent is the knee meniscus, has very few blood vessels through it. It derives its nutrients from three sources; the vessels of the synovial membrane, the synovial fluid, and the blood vessels of the underlying marrow cavity.

Therefore, if this structure is damaged, it will not regenerate. If it is surgically excised, new fibro cartilage will replace it. However, it does not attain quite the same quality, shape and structure as the original articular cartilage.

TENDONS AND LIGAMENTS

These are formed of white tissue which develops in response to tensile strains in situations where strength is required without rigidity or extensibility.

When a tendon or ligament is severed or partly injured, fibroblasts grow in from the surrounding connective tissue and arrange themselves on strands of fibrin, which form as the outcome of the preliminary aseptic inflammation induced by the injury and extend from one stump to the other. Subsequently, these cells become elongated and form collagen fibres which, as usual, are fine at first and gradually become thicker.

The blood supply to ligaments and tendons is poor, so healing is slow, much slower than more copiously supplied tissues such as muscle.

The parallel alignment of fibres in a tendon and their orientation along the direction of maximum tension exerted by the associated muscle suggests that tension playing over the region of regeneration determines the structure of the new tissue.

MUSCLE

The repair of damage to skeletal muscle involves two separate processes. The first is the formation of non-contractile collagenous fibres, the second depends on the capacity of the muscle tissue for regeneration.

Following injury, the tissue is infiltrated by macrophages. These cells are converted to fibroblasts which proliferate rapidly in the damaged area. These fibroblasts secrete a soluble protein percursor of collagen and, in their mature form, the cells remain in the tissue as fibrocytes. The process of maturation is accompanied by a shortening of the fibrocytes, leading to the tendency of muscle wounds to heal short.

The biological key to healing of muscles, however, is the knowledge that muscle cells do regenerate. Experimental work with animals has demonstrated that skeletal muscle possesses a high capacity for regeneration. Researchers have found that when complete animal muscles were removed, minced into small pieces, and replaced in their original sites, progressive regeneration took place during the succeeding weeks, spreading through the muscle mass, which then re-attached to the existing tendon stumps. The original fibres degenerated and disappeared and cross-striations began to appear in the new developing fibres. The contractile property of the muscle also gradually returned, the first response being observed about seven to eight days after the operative procedure.

Although functional regrowth of the regenerating muscle occurred, complete recovery in terms of strength was not achieved. It was found that the new muscle contained relatively few fibres, and large amounts of connective tissue, so that the total tension that the muscle was capable of producing was therefore less than that of normal muscles.

Although these results were obtained in animals, workers in the field tend to agree that there is little doubt that similar results generally would apply to human skeletal muscle.

Sporting injuries are rarely as gross as those mentioned in these experiments; however, the same type of healing procedure (and therefore the same limitations), will take place in varying degrees depending on the amount of damage to the muscle or its component structures.

Occasionally, a serious complication of muscle injuries during healing is the development of myositis ossificans. This ossification process is due to the invasion of the haematoma formed at the time of the injury by osteoblasts (cells which form bone) which are probably derived from the damaged periosteum, the outer coating of bone. Maturation of these cells leads to the formation in the muscle of an open network of bone, and if not properly managed, can seriously impair future function. (Refer to "Haematoma", chapter 7, "Thigh injuries".)

SCAR TISSUE AND PATIENT MANAGEMENT

The repair of soft tissue damage in the human organism is effected by non-specific connective tissue composed very largely of the fibrous protein collagen.

Observers have no hesitation in concluding that basically the same type of connective scar tissue develops at the end of healing, irrespective of the tissue injured, whether it be skin, tendon, ligament or muscle.

This scar tissue is diminished in many of the fitness parameters of the tissue that it is replacing, particularly in the two important components of flexibility and strength. Other constituents of fitness, such as agility, co-ordination, endurance, speed and power will be affected to varying degrees. The athlete, therefore, when returning from injury, may be disadvantaged in skills requiring these facilities.

1 MANAGEMENT OF SCAR TISSUE RIGIDITY AND LOSS OF EXTENSIBILITY

One of the drawbacks of scar tissue is its rigidity and tendency to contract and deform; see figure 2.3.

Researchers, in their series of experiments on rat skins, showed that a sutured wound was slightly more extensible than a tape-closed wound (30 per cent to 42 per cent) when expressed as a percentage of its original length, but neither showed as much extensibility as unwounded skin (56 per cent). This result was found at about 100 days, although there seemed to be very little recovery after 40 days.

Bioengineers have shown that extensibility is as important functionally as strength. For a muscle to attain full power it must

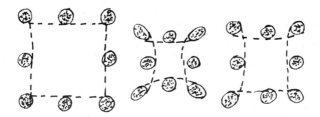

Figure 2.3 A schematic drawing demonstrating wound contraction after a square was excised from a guinea pig's skin. At ten days, contraction is most marked. After ten months, the resultant scar has expanded owing to collagen remodelling and intussusceptive growth (after E. Peacock and W. Van Winkle, *Surgery and Biology of Wound Repair*, W.B. Saunders 1970).

be fully stretched before contraction. Many workers have drawn attention to the fact that fibrosis and scarring in muscle injuries leads to tethering and functional shortening. Similarly, it has been claimed that during the healing of muscles, if the muscle is kept in a shortened or relaxed position, the resultant scar tissue will form a short bridge which may tear again when the muscle is fully stretched out for the first time on the track.

It is important, therefore, that stretching exercises be instituted *early* if normal flexibility is to be regained. For example, by actively stretching haematomas (bruises) of the thigh to their fullest pain-free extent, adhesion formation was limited and the thigh muscles were able to return to the pre-injury range of motion. Since then, many authors have emphasised and confirmed this fact. This principle is supported by further research which has noted that pressure and tension ameliorate contraction caused by scarring.

The essence of all active treatment of muscle injuries in trained athletes is that active rehabilitation of the muscle can be commenced during healing. In other words, one does not need to wait for full anatomical healing before starting to retrain the muscle. The retraining can be started, gradually at first, during the healing period.

This same principle applies also to ligamentous and tendon injuries. Sports medicine authorities have stressed that if exercises are not commenced to restore gradually the full range of movement after an injury to the ankle joint, a chronic sprained ankle may result, with associated pain, swelling and movement limitations.

This principle is substantiated when one considers the physiologic healing process itself. Collagen fibres cannot contract. However, they can be stretched, because after injury they may be woven into a random mesh, kinked or coiled. Stretching is merely a straightening or re-orientation of the fibres, without a change in their dimensions. Further, researchers agree that the most important way of controlling contraction is by a range of carefully planned movement exercises. These serve the purpose of remodelling the developing collagen. Since there is a high collagen turnover in new wounds, properly applied physical therapy can remodel the scar tissue. Range of motion exercises ignore fibroblast pull and concentrate on remodelling the collagen as it is laid down.

It is important that exercises are carried out *within limits of pain*. It is emphatically stated that whatever hurts is wrong; whatever does not hurt is right. Pain, indeed, is nature's guideline, and if stretching exercises are pushed too far into this painful range, obviously more soft tissue damage may result leading to further scar formation.

It has been shown that the best way to lengthen connective tissue structures permanently, including scar formations, without compromising their structural integrity is prolonged, low-intensity stretching at elevated tissue temperatures, cooling the tissue before releasing the tension.

Further discussions on methods of improving range of joint mobility are continued in chapter 5, "Rehabilitation of the Injured Athlete".

2   *TENSILE STRENGTH OF SCAR TISSUE*

When considering the strength of wounds, it is of particular importance to consider the role played by collagen. When the body requires tensile strength, collagen is the substance used. Thus tendons and ligaments are comprised largely of collagen, and liver and muscle have low collagen content. It is now known that there are at least four types of collagen. The most common, type I, makes up the majority of skin, bone and tendon, while type II collagen is found in *cartilage*. Type III is found in embryonic tissues and the cardiovascular system, while type IV makes up basement membrane. Of interest to the problems of wound repair, evidence suggests that although tendon collagen is normally type I, it is replaced by type III during repair. Furthermore, other studies suggest that type III collagen may form a scaffolding in early dermal wound healing which is later replaced by type I collagen. The implications are, of course, that such alterations in collagen types may be extremely important in normal healing and in the pathogenesis of abnormal wound repair.

Cross-linking and remodelling of collagen fibres may require up to six months or a year to complete (the longer time being observed in essentially fibrous tissue such as fascia) and it is important to appreciate that the apparently well healed wound is still a weak and brittle structure five months after injury. Tensile strength at that time is known to be only about 10 per cent of the normal value.

In fact, it has been shown by scanning electon microscopy that *scar tissue is never as strong as the tissue it replaces*.

In their experiments on rat skin wounds, workers in the field tested the mean tensile strength of tape-closed wounds and sutured wounds. Both gained strength with time, but the tape-closed wound gained significantly more than the sutured. By 150 days, it had recovered 90 per cent of the strength of the unwounded skin, whereas sutured ones only regained 70 per cent.

When considering the strength of injured tissues, it has been emphasised that the ability of a wound to resist rupture should be assessed from its energy absorption capabilities. Wounded skin only slowly gains its capacity to absorb energy. After ten days, the wound has recovered 4 per cent of its unwounded value and after 150 days, it has recovered only just over 50 per cent of its original value.

A similar result was found by researchers when reporting on a study of surgically repaired Achilles tendon ruptures. The strength and power of the musculotendinous unit were evaluated with a Cybex II isokinetic unit, the evaluations being performed from 6 to 144 months post-operatively. The repaired tendon had a 16.5 per cent loss of plantar flexion strength and 17.5 per cent loss of plantar flexion power. The early repairs had a smaller loss of strength and power than late repairs.

To compensate for this lack of strength in the scar tissue, it is important that the *sportsperson* participates in an intensive, well-planned strengthening program.

When the injury has occurred in a musculotendinous unit, the athlete undergoes a training program to develop strength, power and endurance of the unit. Similarly, for an injured joint structure, the damaged structures plus the muscles controlling the joint must be strengthened. It is a common clinical observation that overload appears to strengthen ligaments, and this is supported by experimental evidence. Many researchers have now shown by exercising rats and dogs (running and swimming) that there is a close relationship between the strength of the knee ligaments and the mechanical stress to which they are subjected. Other workers have also found that the ligament strength of animals which were exercised was greater than that of those on sedentary programs.

Further, of direct importance to wound healing potential, it has been shown that the strength of repaired ligaments in normal rats and dogs is increased with exercise training and decreased with immobilisation. Thus, it is quite clear that a tissue is as strong as the load that is placed on it.

Methods of overloading strength, power and endurance are discussed in chapter 5, "Rehabilitation of the Injured Athlete".

CHRONIC SCARRING SYNDROME

One aspect of wound healing that deserves special attention, particularly from physiotherapists, is the identification and consequential management of a chronic soft tissue injury; "chronic" generally referring to a condition of more than 6 weeks' duration.

These conditions present a particular consistent pattern of symptoms. The patient will complain of a dull ache or toothache type of pain in the affected area whilst immobile, such as after sitting for a while, or lying in bed, particularly first thing in the morning. The injured area will also ache if exposed to cold, such as during cold weather, or when working in a refrigerated room, or close to an air conditioner. The pain can then be relieved temporarily by heat application and/or exercise. For example, a ligament injury to the ankle may be painful at the commencement of a training session, but after a heat treatment and a thorough warm-up, the pain decreases and may even disappear. However, after training, when the patient cools down, the ache will return. Further, if the injury is one strongly influenced by the force of gravity (such as the abovementioned ankle injury), it may become swollen after the session as well.

These symptoms only become obvious in the later stages of healing, and indeed may still be a considerable problem many months after the original occurrence.

Accordingly, the authors note that these symptoms will *permanently* disappear only after the patient has undergone a very specific exercise program, deliberately designed to stretch and strengthen and regain all parameters of fitness of the damaged structure or structures.

It is the authors' hypothesis that these symptoms may be attributed largely to ischaemia which occurs as a result of contraction due to scarring. The initial examination must carefully scrutinise and evaluate the ranges of movement of joints, muscles and tendons of the damaged area. This testing will always reveal a degree of limitation of flexibility of the structure concerned.

Ischaemia refers to a reduction in the total blood flow in the area supplied by an artery. It is a matter of common clinical experience that haemorrhage occurs in the majority of soft tissue injuries because of damage to arteries. The extent of damage depends on the severity of the wound and there can be no doubt that the consequential fibrous tissue can disrupt the vascularity of a structure further. The duration of ischaemia following occlusion of an artery will depend on the rate at which the collateral circulation develops. With myocardial ischaemia, for example, it is known that it may not reach its full value for up to two months.

It has been shown earlier, in the section "Scar tissue and patient management" in this chapter, how scar tissue can contract and deform. It is therefore hypothesised that as scar fibres kink and coil, they disrupt circulation, which in turn causes ischaemia and consequential pain. It is well recognised and documented that ischaemia can, in fact, cause pain.

When considering the reaction of heat on soft tissue, it has been shown that temperature has a significant influence on the mechanical behaviour of connective tissue under tensile stress. As tissue temperature rises, stiffness decreases and extensibility increases. The mechanism behind this thermal transition is still uncertain, but it is thought that intermolecular bonding becomes partially destabilised, enhancing the viscous flow properties of the collagenous tissue.

As both heat application and exercise can produce a temperature rise, it is suggested that this effect also allows the circulation to improve, thus lessening ischaemic pain.

Further, it is suggested that when a specific stretching program is followed (as specified in chapter 5 on "Rehabilitation"), thus more permanently reorganising the scar fibres and allowing the circulation to become normal, the painful symptoms will disappear permanently.

SUMMARY

This chapter has discussed the phenomena of wound healing, and examined the nature and properties of scar tissue in relation to the rehabilitation of the athlete. It has looked at the process of inflammation and repair and considered the effects of various influential factors on the resultant scar tissue. Further, it has stressed the necessity for controlled stretching to manage scar tissue rigidity, and the importance of a planned strengthening, endurance and power exercise program to compensate for the loss of these parameters in the healing scar.

Finally, of particular interest for physiotherapists, this chapter has researched the probable causes of specific pain experienced in the later stages of wound healing and suggested that ischaemia may be the cause, and that an appropriate prescribed exercise program may be the answer.

PART II
MANAGEMENT OF INJURIES

3
IMMEDIATE MANAGEMENT
OF THE INJURED PLAYER

This chapter is concerned with the immediate management of injury in the field or at the site of play. It outlines procedures to assist decision making on whether an athlete should return to play, or not. Emergency procedures are discussed for when an athlete's life may be in danger and also to cater for most common injuries. A section on the immediate treatment of soft tissue injuries is included, with a section on bandaging and a recommended first aid kit. Topics covered are:
* on the field management;
* emergency procedures;
* immediate treatment of soft tissue injuries;
* bandaging and wound dressings; and
* recommended first aid equipment.

ON THE FIELD MANAGEMENT

Possibly the most difficult phase of injury prevention is encountered when a first aider is called to a player who has sustained an injury and a decision has to be made on whether the player should retire from the game. A methodical system to manage injuries on the field is virtually in the palm of your hand if the mnemonic P.A.L.M. is memorised:

P   Avoid PANIC
A   ASSESS, then ASK or A.B.C.
L   LOOK
M   Test MOVEMENT

P.A.L.M.

Avoid Panic

The most important single thing to remember in this situation is not to panic. Hurry to the patient, but don't be pressured into giving a hasty decision by an excited crowd, a frustrated player, or an enthusiastic referee.

A calm, accurate assessment of the situation may often avoid a player's premature removal from the ground, or prevent him from playing on with an injury that could be seriously worsened by doing so – *do not panic*.

Assess, Ask or A.B.C.

On reaching the injured player, quickly assess the situation.

If the player is unconscious, remember the A.B.C. for unconscious patients – check airways, breathing and circulation. (See the section on "Emergency procedures", "Unconsciousness".) If possible, an unconscious player should be seen by a doctor before being moved.

If the player is conscious, and the problem is not immediately obvious (such as a dislocated shoulder), *ask* what is the matter, but don't immediately touch. Don't drag players to their feet before anything else is done – this may have disastrous results. If the player is not sure exactly what may have happened, ask the referee, other players or even bystanders. Ask leading questions to help gain an accurate description of the history of the injury. This can be a tremendous help in formulating a diagnosis and thereby guiding your decision making. For example, once you ascertain that the player has hurt an ankle, ask if the athlete fell or was kicked. Did he or she hear or feel a crack? Was the athlete moving, and if so, in what direction, and how did he or she fall? These sorts of questions will help you to reach a positive diagnosis.

Look Without Manhandling

It is possible to make a further assessment of the extent of the injury simply by looking. Look for signs that will help to localise and identify the condition, such as swelling, bleeding, abnormal deviations of limbs, the colour of the patient and the injured area, and the position the player was in when you arrived.

If the injured area is swollen at the time of this early examination, it is an indication of rapid tissue bleeding. Swelling from normal inflammatory processes may take up to two hours to become obvious. If the injured limb has turned white or pale, it is an indication of arterial blockage, whilst if it changes to blue, it means the venous circulation is impeded or blocked. Any of these conditions will generally necessitate immediate removal from the field of play.

Test Movement

The player should first test movement; then you do this. Injured athletes should be encouraged to remain quiet until they have demonstrated their ability to move all limbs *unassisted*. Nothing should be done which tends to increase pain, as it almost certainly will increase damage. If they can move all limbs comfortably, they can be encouraged to stand *by their own efforts*. If athletes have to be helped to their feet, they are not going to get back into the game any sooner and may damage themselves further.

If the player can't move a particular limb unassisted, gently try to move it yourself to find what may be limiting the motion. If this increases the pain, the player should be brought from the field to the sideline, where a more searching examination may reveal the full problem (see chapter 4, the section "Signs and symptoms").

From these remarks, it is clear that the first aider's role on the ground is basically one of finding out. If athletes are able to continue playing by their own efforts, no treatment should be necessary. The application of the "magic sponge" serves only to refresh players and give them a minute's breather. That, coupled with a knowledge that they are not seriously injured, allows them to make a "remarkable" recovery.

If, on the other hand, the player has to be removed from the field, active treatment should be started immediately. Treatment may consist of applying emergency procedures or following the suggested techniques for immediate management of soft tissue injury. In-depth discussions of these topics are presented further on in this chapter.

To sum up, in managing injuries on the field, bear in mind the four points contained in the mnemomic *P.A.L.M.*: avoid PANIC; ASSESS the situation, then ASK about the problem or apply A.B.C.; LOOK – don't manhandle; and then test MOVEMENT – the injured person first, then you.

EMERGENCY PROCEDURES

UNCONSCIOUSNESS

Upon reaching the injured athlete, check to see whether he or she is conscious. Shake the patient's shoulder gently and shout "Are you all right?" If there is no response, quickly assess the situation to establish any obvious causes, such as strangulation by a tight or torn jersey and then remove any such causes. Remember the A.B.C. for unconscious players — airways, breathing and circulation — and you will do much to save the athlete's life.

1   Airways

Check to see that the airways are clear and unobstructed. Mud, foreign material or even the player's own tongue may be preventing air getting into the lungs. Roll the patient into the recovery position (fig. 3.4) on his/her side, and remove the obstruction. At the same time, put the head in maximum backward tilt, while supporting the jaw at the point of the chin or at the angle of the jaw.

2   Breathing

If the airways are clear, but breathing has stopped or is becoming weaker, begin artificial resuscitation immediately; see figure 3.1.

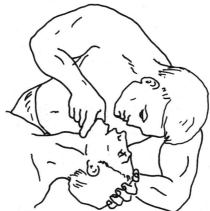

Figure 3.1 Mouth-to-mouth resuscitation (Expired Air Resuscitation — E.A.R.).

a. Maximum head tilt is applied.
b. The jaw is lifted and supported, and the patient's mouth is opened slightly.
c. The operator then takes a deep breath, opens his/her mouth wide, places it firmly over the patient's mouth and blows, and, at the same time, observes the rise of the patient's chest. The operator seals the patient's nose with his/her cheek.
d. After inflation, the operators turns his/her head towards the patient's chest, placing an ear near the patient's face, listening and feeling for the air leaving the patient's mouth and nose. At the same time, the operator observes the patient's chest falling as the air is expired.
e. The operator breathes at the rate of 10 to 15 breaths a minute.

If the mouth has been badly damaged (by a kick, perhaps), mouth-to-nose resuscitation must be instituted. Keep checking on the colour of the patient's lips; pink is healthy, blue means a diminished oxygen supply.

3 Circulation

Feel for the carotid pulse on the side of the neck under the sternomastoid muscle. Do not test this continuously, however, as there is a chance of reducing blood flow to the brain. Meanwhile, if the radial pulse can be felt, it is safe to feel that continuously. Study figure 3.2.

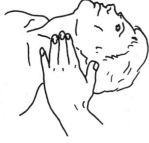 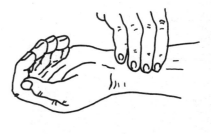

a. Carotid pulse — feel under the sternomastoid muscle.

b. Radial pulse — feel with three or four fingers — not the thumb. Note the radial artery is on the thumb side of the wrist.

Figure 3.2   Locating pulses.

If the pulse is absent, the patient is in a state of cardiac arrest. Begin external cardiac compression immediately in an effort to restart the heart.

When the player has regained both circulation and breathing, leave him or her in the coma position shown in figure 3.4, so that excretion, saliva, vomit, and so on, can drain from the mouth and not obstruct the air passages. It is essential to monitor the circulation and breathing continually.

SPINAL INJURIES

Injuries to the spinal complex are fairly common in sport, particularly contact sport, and may range from minor bruising

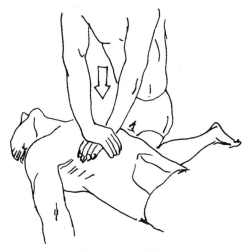

Figure 3.3 External Cardiac Compression (E.C.C.).

a. Place the heel of your hand over the lower half of the patient's breastbone (sternum); your upper hand locks around your wrist, one hand over the other.
b. Compression should move the sternum 4-5 cm, and should be once every 3 to 4 seconds (average about 70 to 80 beats per minute).
c. E.C.C. should be combined with E.A.R. (resuscitation). Synchronise 8 lung inflations with 60 compressions of the heart (2:15 ratio).
d. Return of pulse should be checked every two minutes.

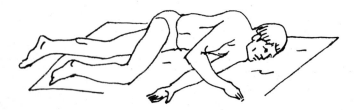

Figure 3.4 The coma or recovery position.

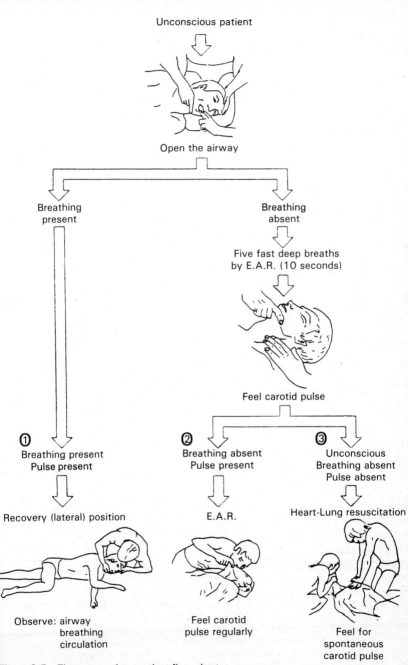

Figure 3.5 The unconscious patient flow chart.
Source: Surf Lifesaving Association of Australia.

to severe damage. Injury may occur to the structures which make up the vertebral column (namely, vertebral bones, discs, ligaments, muscles or nerves), or to the spinal cord, or both. Detailed management of injuries involving the soft tissue of the vertebral column is dealt with in chapter 8.

In *all* cases, however, it is important to allow the player to rise unassisted from the lying position into a seated position, and then to stand up. Assistance should *not* be given, as rough handling in the case of a serious injury can be disastrous. If athletes are unable to get up by their own efforts because of pain or because they find movement difficult, they are best removed from the ground quickly by stretcher with the minimum amount of disturbance in position.

If the player is unconscious as well, roll him or her *gently* onto the side, and ensure breathing is unobstructed. It is most important to assume that an unconscious patient with a head injury may also have a neck injury, and such a patient should be treated accordingly. If the athlete has to be rolled or lifted, ensure that the spine is supported at all times by at least four people. The *Jordan frame* is an excellent means of lifting an unconscious player, provided that the head is properly supported by a third person, or else tied in place with bandages. The Jordan frame is a lifting device and should not be used as a stretcher.

People with injured spines are usually conscious, however, and can tell you if they are unable to feel or move. Ideally, in this

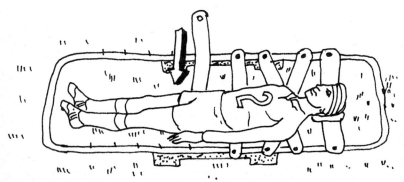

Figure 3.6 Jordan frame; note, if unconscious, the patient should always be kept in the recovery position, in case of vomiting.

a. Place Jordan frame over the injured player.
b. Place the support strips in position.
c. Support the head (to prevent rolling).

situation, the ambulance should be driven onto the field and the patient carefully transferred.

In the changing rooms or ambulance, once the protective muscle spasm has been relieved, many neck and back injuries will recover fairly rapidly. Those which do not recover require medical attention.

Signs of Spinal Cord Damage

The complete spinal cord injury usually shows total loss of function and muscle tone beneath the site of injury as the cord has been interrupted. There is also complete sensory loss (no feeling), and a spinal injury negates reflexes. In the male, an erection is an extremely bad sign, as it almost invariably means the lesion is complete.

The breathing pattern may be altered, as the secondary muscles of breathing may be paralysed. Breathing with the abdomen alone (diaphragmatic breathing) suggests spinal injury.

However, keep in mind that these signs may also appear in a less serious case due to the initial shock and trauma to the spinal column. If no serious lesion has occurred to the spinal cord, the symptoms may be reversible as the swelling and pressure subside.

In all cases of back injury, the player should pass urine into a bottle before leaving the rooms so that the possible presence of blood in the urine is not overlooked. This simple procedure will ensure *early* detection of kidney damage.

FRACTURES

A fracture may be a complete break in the continuity of a bone, or it may be an incomplete break or crack. The cause may be sudden direct violence, such as from a blow, or stress being transmitted along a bone, as when the ankle twists, fracturing the tibia. It is also possible to fatigue a bone by continued repetitive overuse and in this way cause a stress fracture.

Basically, there are two categories of fractures: closed or open.

A fracture is "closed" or "simple" when there is no communication between the site of fracture and the exterior of the body. An "open" or "compound" fracture occurs when the external air is in communication with the fracture. Figure 3.7 shows both closed and open fractures.

Fractures are further divided into various types. Some of the more common ones occurring in sport are shown in figure 3.8, (a)–(g).

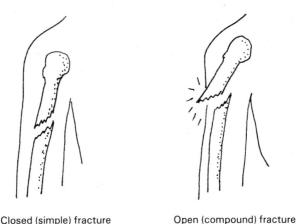

Closed (simple) fracture   Open (compound) fracture

Figure 3.7   Closed and open fractures.

Symptoms

Symptoms which should arouse suspicion of a fracture include pain, swelling at the seat of injury, bruising, and loss of power and movement. However, if these are the *only* symptoms, an X-ray is needed for confirmation. The *only* three features which give unmistakable evidence of a fracture are abnormal mobility, deformity and a grating sound (crepitus). If any of these three symptoms are present, do not proceed with any more diagnostic tests, particularly ones involving movement.

Treatment

If in doubt, do not move the patient until qualified help arrives, particularly if there is a suspicion of a fractured vertebra or other spinal damage.

The application of ice packs at this stage can do no harm and may also ease the pain. The patient should be made as comfortable as possible. Any open wounds should be covered with a clean dressing, and the suspected fracture site should be immobilised as soon as possible.

Generally, a sling for the upper limb and a splint for the lower limb are the best means of support. When splinting, remember to immobilise the joints above and below the suspected fracture site. Then arrange for urgent medical attention. If a patient has

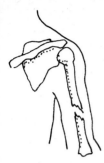

a. Longitudinal fracture (bone splits along its length).

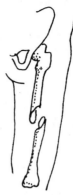

b. Spiral fracture (a rotary force is applied to a long bone).

c. Depressed fracture (it occurs in flat bones, cheek, skull).

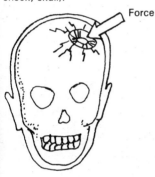

Force

d. Comminuted fracture (three or more bone fragments).

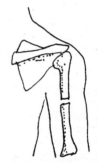

e. Transverse fracture (a direct outside blow causes a fracture at right angles).

f. Contrecoup fracture (a fracture which is found on the side opposite the part where the actual trauma occurred).

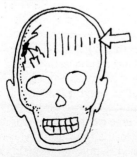

Force

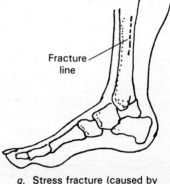

Fracture line

g. Stress fracture (caused by overuse).

Figure 3.8 Types of fractures.

to be moved with a fractured limb, firmly support the limb while applying longitudinal traction; that is, steadily pull the damaged ends of the bone apart along the direction of the limb, to ease the pain.

Note — if there is too much unnecessary movement, it is possible for a splintery broken bone to complicate matters and damage both nerve endings and blood vessels. In its worst form, this complication may lead to necrosis (death) to the injured limb. Take care — if you have any reason to suspect a fracture may be present, do not allow a player to continue in the game under any circumstances.

BLEEDING

External

The normal clotting mechanism of the blood will control most bleeding, caused externally from cuts, abrasions and so on, within about five minutes. If a more drastic open wound occurs (which, incidentally, is rare in sport), immediate *direct pressure* using a sterile compress is the most effective way to control excessive bleeding. The patient should be rested, and an injured limb should be raised. Do not use a tourniquet unless medical help is only fifteen minutes away or unless the bleeding is profuse.

Internal

This may occur from a blow to any of the internal organs, such as liver, spleen or kidneys. The first obvious symptom will be shock, and the patient should be managed accordingly.

Do not give patients fluids, as they may need surgery.

SHOCK

A patient will exhibit symptoms of shock when plasma and oxygen (blood supply) is denied to certain organs and tissues, and when there is a decreased venous blood return to the heart. This may happen, for example, if a player has received a hard blow resulting in extreme internal bleeding or a severe fracture. It may also occur from dehydration or illness.

Athletes suffering from shock become extremely pale and will probably break out in a cold sweat, although they can be shivering. They may complain of severe abdominal pain, even though they have not been struck in the abdomen, and want to vomit. The abdomen may feel extremely hard and distended and the pulse may be rapid and weak.

Remove the athlete from the ground immediately and call a physician. These signs may mean serious trouble and prompt action could well save a life.

In all accidents involving shock symptoms, the general principles to follow can be remembered with the help of the mnemonic W.A.R.

W   WARMTH; use a rug
A   AIR; provide cool, fresh air and plenty of it (oxygen if necessary and available)
R   RAISE the legs

However, in severe cases of shock, where there has been great blood loss, too much warmth may be detrimental, as it may cause the peripheral blood vessels to dilate. The body will need to constrict these blood vessels naturally to maintain blood pressure, so in these cases it may be better *not* to cover the patient with a rug.

HEAT INJURIES

Heat exhaustion, leading to heat stroke, can occur when the body cannot conduct excessive heat from its system. It occurs more quickly in people who are not properly conditioned for their sport, in people who are not acclimatised and in people who are overweight. The risk of heat injury will be greater if the sport or training is carried out on a particularly hot day or in a confined area with no fresh air circulation, such as in a squash court or gymnasium.

Heat Exhaustion

The warning symptoms of heat exhaustion include:
- excessive sweating;
- elevated body temperature;
- headache;
- nausea, vomiting;
- fatigue.

Heat Stroke

Without treatment, heat exhaustion will lead on to heat stroke. Further symptoms will include:

- dry, hot skin, no sweating when you would expect profuse sweating;
- high body temperature, over 41 degrees C;
- seizures, coma, unconsciousness;
- rapid breathing;
- vomiting, stomach cramps;
- pilo-erection (goose pimples) and chilling, shivering.

Treatment

The treatment for heat injury is aimed at reducing the body temperature and replacing lost fluids. Place the athlete in the shade, with airways open and clear for breathing. Your patient should then be sponged with ice or cold water and fanned vigorously, and at the earliest convenient time, he or she should be encouraged to drink water, steadily. When it is suspected that athletes have heat stroke they should be removed to a hospital as soon as possible.

Prevention

General principles for the prevention of heat injury are given here:
1 Fluids and electrolytes (body salts) must be replaced regularly during prolonged physical activity. It is important to have "water stations" at least every three to four kilometres for road training or long distance competition. An athlete should drink an adequate amount of water at least 15 minutes before training or playing. However, if glucose or sugar is added, this may slow down the absorption rate considerably, so this mixture should be drunk at least two to three hours beforehand, then regular amounts of fluid taken in small doses. A footballer should have a drink through the game as well as at half-time.
2 The athlete should become acclimatised to the heat. It takes at least four to seven days to become acclimatised. This is important when competing in a different climate.
3 Athletes should not compete in endurance events unless they are appropriately trained.
4 Sensible, cool clothing should be worn when training, not raincoats or plastic vests. If athletes are training to lose weight, they must not believe that because they are sweating they are effectively losing calories. Any weight reduction by fluid loss will be restored within 12 hours by drinking. Wearing heavy tracksuits will simply prevent the sweat from reaching the outside environment and doing the job it was designed to do;

cooling the body by evaporation. Wearing heavy and non-porous clothing is a dangerous practice.

5 Educate the athlete to recognise the symptoms of heat injury.

CRAMPS

A cramp is a strong, continual contraction affecting a muscle. It can be extremely painful, depending on the force and duration of the contraction.

Cramps appear to be the result of inadequate nutrition to a muscle. This effect can be caused by different factors:

- The diet may be inadequate. It is thought the most important salts involved in muscle contraction are potassium and magnesium as well as *normal* salt. It appears that potassium is lost in large amounts during hard exercise, and this deficiency can be remedied by eating adequate fruits, vegetables and grains. It is recommended that you do not take salt tablets routinely, except on a physician's advice.
- There may be a lack of general or specific fitness, thus denying the muscle ready adequate nutrition.
- Garters or clothing may be too tight and restrictive.
- Sustained muscular contractions can be preventing a normal blood supply (as in the bent-knee stance of snow-skiing).

Treatment

The most common muscles to sustain cramps are those in the calf, so obviously, remove any restricting garters and clothing first.

The muscle should be stretched, gently, in the opposite direction to that in which it normally contracts. A gentle massaging action over the muscle may help to relieve the spasm, as may thumb pressure over the middle of the muscle bulk. If the cramp continues, the player should be removed from the field and an ice pack applied to the muscle.

KICK IN ABDOMEN OR TESTICLES

If a player is merely "winded", recovery will be much quicker if he or she is left alone with no treatment except encouragement. Do not "pump" the legs or force the knees into the abdomen, as this may only make the situation worse (because of fractured ribs or bleeding into the abdominal cavity).

Abdomen

Loosen the player's pants, and sit the injured player up, keeping the hips flexed (bent). While standing behind and supporting the player with your knees, place your fingertips below the ribcage and lift as he or she breathes in; then allow the abdomen to drop. Repeat this procedure until the player resumes normal breathing.

Be on the lookout for internal bleeding and symptoms of shock. It is wise to inform the patient of shock symptoms as a slow bleed may not become noticeable until some hours after the event, and the athlete must be aware of any possible complications.

Testicles

The initial problem caused by a severe blow to the testicles may be an inability to breathe because of spasm of the diaphragm and breathing muscles from pain. Use the method described above for the abdomen to restart normal breathing.

As with the abdomen, be wary of slow bleeding, in this case into the scrotum. The testicles may need to be supported in a cotton-wool sling if they do become painful and swollen (fig. 3.9). The application of ice will help to ease the pain and control bleeding. However, if swelling from haemorrhaging continues, the player should see a physician urgently.

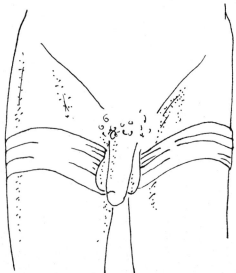

Figure 3.9   Scrotal sling.

HEAD AND FACIAL INJURIES

Head Injuries—Including Brain

Trauma to the head may cause:
- injury to the soft tissues;
- fracture of the skull;
- injury to the brain.

Injury to soft tissues

As the head is copiously supplied with blood, lacerations and cuts bleed freely, but are easily controlled by firm pressure.

Fracture of the skull

Fractures may result from direct violence, for example, being struck by a cricket ball, a boot or a hockey stick, or from striking the ground. They may be exposed to the open air (compound fractures), or they may be closed. Coincidental damage to the brain or the blood vessels surrounding the brain gives varying grades of concussion and/or compression.

In the main, head injuries on the field are relatively minor and, unless there is quite a long period of amnesia, the player can be left alone. If there is a long period of amnesia or the patient is irritable or belligerent, he or she should be removed from the field of play, as more than minor concussion has occurred and the possibility of brain damage should be borne in mind.

Injury to the brain

In any head injury, it is the brain damage that matters most.
Concussion   Concussion may be minor, a blow to the head causing some period of memory loss of time in the game and minor headaches, with fairly rapid recovery. In more serious grades of concussion, where the patient is deeply unconscious, if not watched carefully he or she may swallow false teeth or get airway obstruction as a result of the tongue falling back, which compounds the problems in the nervous system. Whenever a patient is knocked unconscious, the essential treatment is to make sure of a good airway, by placing the person in a suitable posture, or in the coma or recovery position, by loosening clothing around the neck, and by removing mouthguards or other things (dirt, and so on) obstructing the airway through the mouth or nose.

(See "Unconsciousness", this chapter.) Beware of neck and spinal injuries with unconscious players.

Compression   Compression is a higher grade concussion and is due to bleeding taking place inside the cranium, causing pressure on vital cranial tissue. The patient becomes too deeply unconscious to arouse, and the pupil of one eye dilates (becomes larger) and does not react to light. This requires *urgent* medical attention.

General Management of Head Injuries

Head injury patients should be taken immediately to hospital or a doctor if they:

- vomit;
- develop a headache;
- become restless or irritable;
- become drowsy, dizzy or cannot be roused;
- have a fit (convulsion);
- or if anything else unusual occurs.

Until then, they should:

- rest quietly;
- not consume alcohol;
- not drive a vehicle.

They should not train or play again without medical clearance from a doctor.

Eye Injuries

The first thing to determine with eye injuries is whether the injury is slight or grave. If it is slight, the patient can often go back onto the field after minor treatment, for example, the irrigation of mud or the removal of a foreign body from the eye.

To irrigate dirt or foreign material from the eye, lay the patient down, gently hold the eyelids apart with the finger and thumb of one hand, and pour sterile saline (salt) solution, for example, Alcon eye stream solution, in the eye socket from a plastic bag held by the other hand. If a foreign body is still present after the procedure and is not on the clear part of the eye (the cornea), try to dislodge it gently with a cotton-wool-tipped applicator. If the patient still complains of a foreign body sensation after irrigation, the upper lid should be everted (turned back). This is best done by asking the patient to look down, seizing the eyelashes of the upper lid with the finger and thumb, and pulling the lid gently down and turning it back on itself over a blunt pencil or

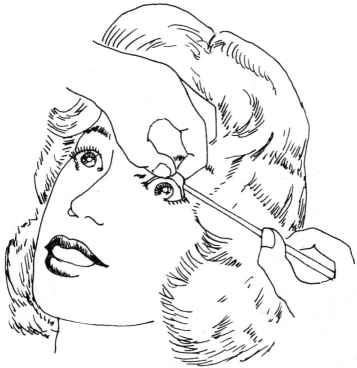

Figure 3.10   Everting the upper eyelid.

glass rod, as in figure 3.10. Sometimes, the foreign body is seen lying on the inner part of the everted lid, from which it can be removed.

Accidents to the eyeball itself, caused either by fists, feet, squash or tennis balls, are best referred to the casualty department of the nearest hospital. If the patient states that he or she has suddenly lost vision ("a curtain went down") the diagnosis may be a detached retina. This, of course, requires urgent medical attention.

Swelling

As the tissues surrounding the eye are very loose, swelling may rapidly close the eye. Ice treatment may be applied; however, do not use heavy packs, or loose ice. It is best to use commercially prepared packs to avoid pressure over the eyeball.

Ear Injuries

The most common injury to the ear is damage to the pinna (the projecting parts), "cauliflower ear" (haematoma of the pinna). This will result from bleeding or infection after trauma to the pinna. The trauma disrupts cartilage and the end result will be a distortion in shape of the pinna.

The immediate treatment is to apply ice with a moderate amount of compression to control the haematoma. However, if the haematoma does develop further, it should be drained (by a doctor) under aseptic conditions at the earliest possible time.

If a foreign body should enter the ear (gravel, stones), it should be removed with the *proper* instruments, *not* forceps;, once again, by a doctor.

Finally, a blow to the ear which causes "ringing" or partial deafness may mean rupture of the eardrum and should be seen immediately by a doctor.

Nose Injuries

A bleeding nose is the most common condition associated with nose injuries. Sit the patient up, instruct him or her to breathe through the mouth, and apply pressure across the bridge of the nose for at least five minutes to allow the the blood to clot. An ice pack will also help to constrict blood vessels and ease the pain. If bleeding cannot be controlled, insert a rolled piece of moistened 2 cm gauze bandage pack into the nostril and seek medical attention.

Fractured noses should be seen by a surgeon as soon as possible after the game.

Teeth Injuries

A comfortably fitting mouthguard, made to fit by a dental surgeon, should be worn at all times in body contact sport. It has been shown that the use of the mouthguard can:
- lessen the chances of concussion from a blow to the jaw;
- lessen the possibility of a broken jaw;
- lessen the possibility of broken and dislodged teeth.

If a tooth is dislodged whole, wash it, keep it in saline solution, and seek dental aid immediately; it may be possible to restore it to the gum.

SKIN INJURIES

Cuts, Abrasions and Grass Burns

Clean the wound thoroughly in the shower first, with soap and water. Then clean it with an antiseptic solution, such as povidone, iodine 10 per cent (commercially, this is known as Betadine, either in solution or as a swabstick). A wound of this nature will heal faster if kept moist, so cover with a dressing such as "Tulle-Gras", an open-weave cotton bandage impregnated with Vaseline, and apply cream medications.

A cut or wound that gapes more than 2 mm should be seen by a medical officer to consider whether or not it requires suturing (stitching).

As many football grounds were once old horse paddocks, it is wise for footballers to have a course of tetanus injections.

Blisters

Clean the surface of the blister with a suitable antiseptic and burst it with a sterile needle (either from a sterile pack or held over an open flame for a minute). After draining the fluid from the blister, cover it with a sterile protective dressing. A doughnut-shaped sponge may be placed around the blister to keep pressure off it. The application of "Second Skin" is an excellent way of allowing continued training with minor blisters.

Prevention

Ensuring that athletic shoes are properly fitting is the most important factor in preventing blisters; second, commence a training program steadily, and at no stage overload too quickly, and thirdly, wear two pairs of socks to lessen the friction of skin on shoes.

Skin is like other tissues; it adapts to increased stress, so time must be allowed for it to accommodate to any increased workload, whether running, rowing or playing tennis.

Tinea

Fungi of all types grow best in conditions of warmth, moisture and darkness, a situation often encountered with sportspeople. The most common fungi are tinea pedis (foot) and tinea cruris (crutch or groin), but it may occur in other areas. The condition will manifest itself as a red, itchy rash which may become infected by continual scratching or irritation. The condition is basically managed by these tactics:

- absolute cleanliness; thorough drying after showers and regular application of talcum powder or tinea powder (obtain from chemist);
- clean clothes at every session of training and play;
- use of a standard fungicide for specific medication.

These are available over the counter.

For resistant or infectious cases, consult the team doctor.

IMMEDIATE TREATMENT OF SOFT TISSUE INJURIES

It must be stressed that speed in applying an active, proven treatment to an injury is one of the most important factors in quick healing. This, of course, applies to all categories of injuries. However, this section deals only with soft tissue injuries and their first aid management. The appropriate way to recognise and treat the emergency situation has been presented earlier in this chapter and management procedures of specific injuries will be discussed in later chapters of this book.

In this context, *soft tissue* refers to ligaments, muscles, tendons, fascia (fibrous tissue), and similar structures and generally will account for the majority of sporting injuries.

The usual signs of tissue reaction to injury are inflammation, haemorrhaging (bleeding), swelling, loss of function, pain and subsequent muscle spasm.

The important aim in the early stages of treatment is to minimise these effects to assist in quicker healing and eventual return to sport. Efforts are directed at preventing and reducing inflammation, stopping the haemorrhaging and relieving pain and spasm. By following the guidelines contained in the mnemonic R.I.C.E. — rest, ice, compression, elevation — you will do as much as any person can do, qualified or otherwise.

R.I.C.E.

Rest

With most injuries, 24-48 hours rest from movement will help to prevent aggravation of the damage and relieve symptoms of shock, pain and spasm. The upper limb should generally be immobilised in a sling and the lower limb supported in either a back slab, compression bandage or splint.

Ice

Ice is applied to an injury for two main reasons: for its effects on circulation in reducing swelling, and for its efficiency as a pain and spasm reliever.

A full discussion on the effects of ice and its application as a treatment modality is presented in chapter 5.

The normal soft tissue injury will slowly swell for at least 24 hours from exudates brought by the circulatory and lymphatic systems as part of the normal healing processes. If the injured part swells grossly within the first half hour after injury, it is usually due to haemorrhaging into the tissue from large ruptured blood vessels. The normal clotting mechanism of the blood will generally stop the bleeding within the first five minutes, but ice treatment, by its vasoconstrictive effect (constriction of blood vessels), will help to prevent and control excess swelling regardless of whether the cause is inflammation or haemorrhage.

However, the most important use of ice at this stage is as an analgesic. After five minutes' application, during which the patient feels cold, then pain, followed by numbness, the ice elevates the pain threshold, increasing the patient's tolerance to pain. This, in turn, facilitates early mobilisation .

Ice Application

Ice can be effectively applied by four different techniques: ice packs, ice massage, ice baths and ice sprays. Ice should never be applied directly to the skin, as it may cause a skin burn. The most effective temperature range for pain relief is within the range of 6 and 10 degrees Celsius. Never use dry ice (frozen carbon dioxide), as its temperature can drop down to below − 43 degrees Celsius, and would obviously cause extensive skin damage.

Place the injured limb, whether the site of injury be knee, hamstring, thigh or even a suspected bone fracture, in a moist towel containing crushed ice; an injured ankle or wrist may be submerged in a bucket of ice water. Leave in this situation for at least 20 to 30 minutes, and repeat this procedure every three to four waking hours for at least 24 to 48 hours. With certain individuals, it may be desirable to leave the ice pack in place for up to three or four hours continuously; there are no dangerous side effects. It is unwise to use heat of any description in this phase, because heat can cause bleeding to start again. Ice will not cause rebleeding.

Compression

A crepe bandage comfortably wrapped around the injury also helps to prevent excess swelling. However, if the bandage is too tight, or if the fluid is allowed to build up, as the limb remains pendant, the bandage may then act as a tourniquet. Keep a check on the extremities for blueness, which indicates a lack of circulation, and numbness, which denotes compression of a nerve. If either occurs, loosen the bandage.

Elevation

As the amount of excess fluid at the site of injury is influenced by the force of gravity, keep an injured limb raised, particularly if the ankle is injured. This enables fluid to drain away from the injury, back into the circulatory and lymphatic systems, thus preventing accumulation, organisation and eventual scarring in the area.

A good technique is to use ice, compression and elevation at the same time.

BANDAGING AND WOUND DRESSING

Bandages and dressings are used to cover and protect a wound and to support injured parts. They are also used to control bleeding and swelling, to prevent or lessen infection and to protect the wound from further injury.

The best dressing for wounds is a sterilised piece of gauze. Avoid touching any part of the gauze which will be in contact with the wound. If using "Tulle-Gras", cut to the size required with a clean pair of scissors and keep in place with a protective bandage.

In sports medicine, the main uses of bandages are:
- to protect a wound — by covering it with a dressing to maintain hygiene;
- to apply compression during the initial stages of an injury in order to control swelling and bleeding;
- to restrict movement — such as immobilising a suspected fracture;
- to afford support — for a weakened or damaged structure, as in a sling.

Other uses are to support sponge pads under the foot and to secure a protective device over a vulnerable area.

PRINCIPLES OF BANDAGING

1 Select the appropriate bandage for the job. Roller bandages are made of many materials: gauze, cotton cloth and elastic wrapping (crepe).
2 Choose the correct width for the particular structure — 2 cm for wrist, thumb and hand; 3 cm for ankle and elbow; 6 cm for knee and shoulder; and 10 cm for thigh and trunk.
3 Hold the bandage with the unrolled portion uppermost and apply the outer surface of the bandage to the part.
4 Bandage from distal to proximal, that is, from the extremity towards the heart, in the direction of the blood returning to the heart through the veins.
5 Unroll only a few centimetres at a time, maintaining even pressure throughout.
6 Overlap the bandage at least half the width of the previous turn.
7 Smooth the bandage as it follows the contour of the skin and limb.
8 Finish off with a straight turn above the part, fold in the end and fasten.
9 Watch for restriction of circulation between the bandage and the extremity. If the bandage is too tight, the circulation and nerve pathways will be impeded. Pink is healthy, but if the extremities turn blue or black or lose their pulse, and also become numb or tingling, release the pressure immediately.

COMMON BANDAGING TECHNIQUES

Circular or Simple Spiral

This is used when the injured part to be bandaged is of relatively uniform thickness, such as a finger, trunk or forearm.

Reverse Spiral

This is used to bandage limbs which are funnel-shaped and not suitable for a simple spiral; e.g. the calf.

Figure-of-eight

Use this technique for joints such as the knee, ankle and elbow.

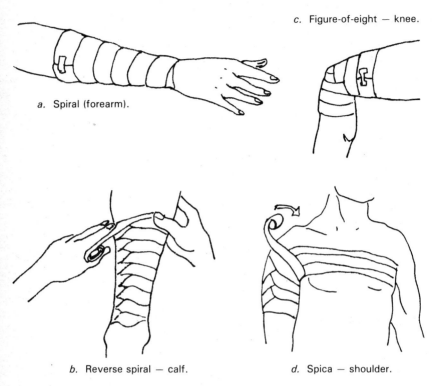

a. Spiral (forearm).

c. Figure-of-eight — knee.

b. Reverse spiral — calf.

d. Spica — shoulder.

Figure 3.11   Common bandaging techniques.

Spica

This is an uneven figure-of-eight used for the thumb, shoulder or hip.

RECOMMENDED FIRST AID EQUIPMENT

(Suggested by the Australian Sports Medicine Federation in *The Sports Trainer*; see the reading list, p. 343.)

Instruments

Forceps, nail clippers (two sizes), safety razor, scissors, sterile needles, tweezers.

Applications

Aerosol dressing, antiseptic powder, methylated spirits, anti-fungal foot powder, Vaseline, antiseptic cream, antiseptic solution, skin toughener, tape adherent, tape remover.

Medications

Aspirin, antacid tablets, nose drops, saline eye drops, saline eye wash.

Dressings

Adhesive first aid strips, cotton buds, cotton wool, elastic adhesive bandage 3.75 cm × 7.5 cm, orthopaedic foam, large absorbent dressings, sterile gauze dressings, sterile gauze pads, eye pads, adhesive dressing tape, paraffin gauze.

Strapping and Bandaging Materials

Cotton bandages – 2.5 cm, 5 cm, 7.5 cm; crepe bandages – 7.5 cm, 10 cm, 15 cm; elastic non-adhesive bandages – 2.5 cm, 5 cm, 7.5 cm; triangular sling; non-stretch adhesive tape – 35 mm and 12 mm; stretch adhesive tape – 2.5 cm and 7.5 cm.

General

Blankets, crutches, first aid book, inflatable splints, Jordan frame, notebook, pen, pencil torch, safety pins, stretcher, clinical thermometer, bucket, ice cold packs, towels (disposable and terry towelling), rubber sponge, coins for telephone.

Bulky Equipment

This should be kept in the dressing or club rooms, in an area that is readily accessible, and includes stretchers, splints, crutches, blankets and medical stock.

4
GENERAL PRINCIPLES FOR THE EVALUATION OF THE INJURED PLAYER

Chapter 4 should be approached with caution by the layperson. It has been written to aid the clinician in assessment procedures. However, it is useful for those involved in the first aid management of injuries to understand the fundamentals of injury assessment. The chapter deals with the general examination and evaluation of a typical limb injury. The approach is classical and methodical, yet experience has shown it to be efficient and practical.

SIGNS AND SYMPTOMS

To make a satisfactory diagnosis, it is necessary to have a full understanding of the significance of the various signs and symptoms produced by the injury. The most commonly occurring signs and symptoms can be summarised broadly:
- pain;
- swelling;
- locking;
- precipitance;
- variations of joint mobility;
- loss of muscular strength;
- muscular atrophy;
- loss of function.

PAIN

The perception of pain is a result of the brain's integration of physiological and psychological mechanisms involving receptors and conductors. The sensory end organs for pain are spread throughout all the tissues of the body, so that basically three kinds of pain are recognised: (a) superficial or cutaneous pain; (b) deep pain from muscles, tendons, joints and fascia; and (c) visceral pain.

The exact causes of pain associated with musculoskeletal injury cannot be stated with any finality. Certainly swelling (from any cause) will increase tissue pressure and can produce pain. The acid ph of the exudate, an accumulation of k + ions, and the presence of chemical mediators like 5-hydroxytryptamine and bradykinin have also all been blamed for the production of pain.

A thorough assessment should cover all aspects and qualities of pain. Throbbing pain at rest, pain on palpation, pain on diagnostic movement and functional movement, and all varying degrees of frequency and intensity add to the overall clinical picture.

SWELLING

Swelling is a clear sign that the body has been injured, although it does not always follow that there will be swelling after injury (for example, a damaged meniscus or cartilage will not always swell). It is important to be able to differentiate between the various qualities of swelling, as the outcome will obviously affect the treatment.

Be aware that the amount of swelling may not parallel the severity of the lesion, as the quantity of observed swelling may vary, being reliant on certain factors. Exercise, immobilisation, elevation and relationship to the force of gravity and tissue tension in the surrounding areas will all affect the amount of swelling resulting from an injury at any given time.

Finally, remember that swelling is never a diagnosis or a condition by itself — it is a symptom. There is no such diagnosis, for instance, as "water on the knee" — you must look for the underlying cause of the "water" or fluid.

LOCKING

This is a symptom most commonly encountered in knee injuries, but other joints can lock. Caution must be taken accepting the patient's interpretation of "locking". He or she may interpret stiffness or lack of movement caused from pain or fluid as meaning locking. True locking is defined as a sudden and complete painful block to extension sustained by the mechanism of knee rotation in flexion. (This symptom is covered further in the section on "Knee injuries", chapter 7).

PRECIPITANCE

Precipitance is the sudden giving way of a joint during function, particularly the knee. It implies a complete inhibition and collapse of the quadriceps action as a result of an internal derangement of the knee joint. It can relate to a wide variety of pathological processes, but the most common underlying lesion is a tear of the posterior segment of the medial meniscus. (This symptom is also further discussed in the section on "Knee injuries", chapter 7.)

VARIATIONS OF JOINT MOBILITY

Virtually any of the symptoms previously discussed, as well as the original causative factor, may have an effect on joint mobility. Pain from any source whatever, the quality of the soft tissue structures after and during the repair process, as well as the mechanical obstruction of fluid in the joint, may all prevent or interfere with joint mobility.

A complete rupture of a ligament or ligaments may allow excessive movements in one or more planes, and may be a diagnostic clue towards an unstable joint.

LOSS OF MUSCULAR STRENGTH

The strength of a muscle is the pulling force or tension that can be exerted during contraction. If the muscle itself has been damaged, and fewer fibres are free to contract, there will obviously be a loss in muscular strength. Damage to muscle fibres and the associated pain and spasm will cause disuse leading to a further diminishing of muscular strength. When joint structures, such as ligaments, are damaged the swelling, pain and muscle spasm will also cause disuse and a reduction in strength of the muscles controlling the joint will be noted. All facets of muscle performance, that is, strength, power and endurance, can be measured on an isokinetic device (for example, a Cybex).

MUSCULAR ATROPHY

It is well recognised that muscular atrophy (or wastage) is a consistent symptom of musculoskeletal injury and is due to the loss of strength, power and endurance of the muscle when injured (disuse atrophy). This situation is obvious in knee joint injuries when marked thigh muscle wastage (quadriceps and hamstrings) is displayed. Muscular atrophy is also evident in nerve injuries, blocking nerve supply to the muscle (for example, deltoid wastage after circumflex humeral nerve damage in the shoulder) and in muscles which have been immobilised in a plaster cast.

LOSS OF FUNCTION

Virtually any of the symptoms previously mentioned, no matter what the cause, or as well as the cause, may lead to a loss in function of the structure which has been damaged.

"Loss of function" is always linked with one or more of these preceding symptoms, although the importance of any other symptoms may be insignificant when compared to the functional disability which follows an injury. In fact, this "loss of function" may be the only reason for seeking treatment. Patients may not have been able to perform a particular skill or movement or participate in certain sports or carry out their normal occupation. Patients may complain that they cannot bend their knee because of pain or swelling, or they cannot walk without limping because the knee may lock, or they cannot swerve or zigzag because the knee keeps "giving way".

Following diagnosis and effective treatment, the patient will eventually regain normal function. Ideally, all symptoms will disappear and the patient should be capable to returning to normal activities of work and sport.

In practice, this standard will alter with the needs of the individual. For instance, a clerical worker may still have slight swelling in his knee after treatment for a medial ligament sprain. This slight swelling may not impair the patient's work duties. However, if the same clerk was a footballer the obvious symptom of swelling would cause a loss of function. Swelling would prevent full flexion and extension of the knee, limiting running speed and pain would be experienced at the knee when stressed in sudden changes of direction.

Clinically, the establishment of full function after injury demands meticulous attention to the intricate details. It involves manual examination, clinical testing on sophisticated devices (for example, the Cybex) and functional testing on the field.

EVALUATION OF THE INJURED PLAYER

Once injured players have been removed from the arena of play or training, they should be showered, if possible, in preparation for a more extensive examination. It is assumed that for any serious injuries requiring life-saving, first aid measures would have been already applied. Once again, a mnemonic is a useful tool in summarising important steps in the evaluation of an injury. So, remain cool and C.A.L.M. and you will be able to handle most limb injuries, soft tissue or otherwise.

C.A.L.M.

    C Clinically assess
    A Ask
    L Look
    M Manually examine

Clinically Assesss

Have the injured player lying comfortably or sitting for best manipulation of limbs. In most cases, the uninjured limb is a mirror image of the injured one, and should be exposed for comparison. Likewise, the area to be examined should be adequately exposed and should be clearly visible with good lighting.

Ask

Establish the history of the injury. In most cases, this will be the most important method of revealing clues to form a diagnosis. Methodically ask questions such as:
  • How did the injury occur?
  • Was it a blow? Did you fall? Were you tackled?
  • How did you land? Twisted or straight? (Try to reconstruct the forces involved and their directions and speed, and calculate where the most stress was likely to be directed.)
  • Did you hear or feel clicking, locking or grating noises? (This is to aid in cartilage and bone damage detection.)
  • When did the injury start to swell? (Swelling within half an hour indicates haemarthrosis—bleeding into the joint. A longer period denotes normal reaction to injury—inflammation.)

- Does the limb lock or give way during use?
- What kind of pain do you feel? (A throbbing pain generally indicates arterial or circulatory involvement; a burning, searing pain with pins and needles will point to nerve damage; and stabbing pain on movement generally denotes ligament or muscle damage. A toothache kind of pain, either when the limb is moved or particularly when at rest, generally means a complication in an old soft tissue injury involving scarring.)

Look

Make a systematic visual examination of the limb, carefully noting the following features:
- Bones. Observe the general alignment and any deformity or unusual shape.
- Soft tissues. Look for contours and shape, comparing both sides; note swelling and muscle wastage.
- Colour and texture of the skin. Look for redness, which indicates inflammation; bluishness, which indicates diminished circulation; or shininess, which generally means nerve damage.

Manually Examine

Manual examination comprises palpation, or feeling, and testing the movement of the limb. When feeling, consider the following points:
1 Temperature. An increase in temperature denotes an increase in local circulation, either from inflammation or from infection. Coolness, of course, indicates decreased blood supply. (Compare the injured limb with the other limb.) However, if the patient has just stopped playing, you must allow for a generally increased body temperature.
2 The bones. Feel for a change in shape, alignment, and for thickening or grating.
3 Soft tissues. This examination is mainly in relation to muscles. Note muscle wastage and muscle spasm. (Spasm is nature's protective device to prevent movement and therefore minimise pain; virtually any injury that elicits pain will cause spasm of its relative muscle group, and this can be a large problem in treatment.) Feel also for the quality of fluids or swellings in joints—a thin, runny fluid denotes normal fluid exudates; a thick, boggy consistency indicates either blood or synovial mucosa thickening (synovial membrane lines the joints); while

thickening of the deeper bony tissues points to an overgrowth, callusing or scarring of an old injury.

4 Tenderness and pain. Try to locate the exact site of pain and relate it to a particular structure.

When testing the movement of a limb, always compare that limb with the other. The aim is to find out what is abnormal with the injured limb. Check for range of movement — limited range of joint movement may be caused by pain from damaged structures, associated muscle spasm, or scarring or adhesions; excessive movement may be caused by muscle paralysis, broken bones, or torn or ruptured tendons or ligaments. Check for crepitus (grating on movement), which may indicate a fracture. Once again, try to localise the pain to a particular anatomical structure. As the limb is moved, note the muscular strength and power and also joint stability. (Remember not to push anything past the limit of pain during examination.)

Included in this movement examination should be a "test of function". How does the injury affect the patient while walking, running, serving in tennis, passing a ball, or carrying out a particular action appropriate to his or her sport? Note any "giving way" of joints, unusual gait patterns, or favouring of limbs. This can be a valuable aid in assessing improvement.

To sum up: (a) *clinically assess*—expose both limbs in good light; (b) *ask*—find out how the injury occurred; (c) *look*—make a visual examination; and (d) *manually examine*—feel for indications, then test movement. If the diagnosis is not immediately clear to you, do not risk a "calculated guess". Refer the patient immediately to a qualified medical officer or physiotherapist for the advantage of clinical experience, plus the chance to use X-rays and blood tests if necessary.

Finally, remember that the patient is a fellow human being who has the same fears and phobias as all of us. A confident, kind, reassuring word during the examination may help to allay any worries that the injury could be terminal or at least could ruin a sporting career.

It is vitally important medically unqualified aiders realise their limitations in injury evaluation. They must refer to the appropriate medical personnel for comprehensive differential diagnosis, based on professional clinical experience and the use of sophisticated equipment and tests, if needed.

A professional examination will consist of a logical and systematic sequence of events leading to the establishment of a diagnosis.

1 History
2 Clinical examination
   (a) Observation
   (b) Palpation
   (c) Measurement
   (d) Movements
3 Radiographic examination
4 Special examination
   (a) Haematological
   (b) Biochemical
   (c) Serological and bacteriological
   (d) Histological
   (e) Electrical.

5
REHABILITATION OF THE INJURED ATHLETE

Rehabilitation begins immediately after injury and continues until the patient is ready to return to his or her sport. He or she must be returned to *full* competitive fitness at the earliest possible moment. This remains the main aim in the rehabilitation of the injured athlete.

The general principles of rehabilitation will be discussed under three major headings:

- *Relief of symptoms*—this section will consider the selection of appropriate modalities to aid in pain relief, reduction of swelling and relaxation of muscle spasm.
- *Regaining all components of fitness of the injured structure*— this section will discuss therapeutic exercise selection to regain flexibility, strength, power, endurance and co-ordination.
- *Regaining functional activity*—this section reinforces the need to develop a "treat and train" attitude when treating sportspeople.

RELIEF OF SYMPTOMS

In order for rehabilitation to proceed effectively, the important symptoms to control immediately are pain, swelling and muscle spasm. Once these reactions have been managed, not only will healing be facilitated, but the patient will also be able to commence a positive therapeutic exercise program.

In the section on "Immediate treatment of soft tissue injuries" in chapter 3, there is a discussion of procedures to follow in the first 24-48 hours. It is essential to relieve pain and associated protective muscle spasm and reduce swelling. As mentioned, the application of the mnemonic R.I.C.E. is a very positive method of achieving these aims.

As swelling is largely caused by the inability of the blood vessels to contain the extra white blood cells and plasma proteins which accumulate at the injury site, the two most effective ways to manage excess swelling are by compression and elevation. The amount of swelling depends on the extent of damage plus the tissue tension of the surrounding structures. For instance, a deep muscle injury may not swell as much as one closer to the surface because of the weaker tension exerted by the skin.

The amount of swelling is also influenced by the force of gravity. If a limb is pendant, fluid (including blood) accumulates in the vicinity of the wound, or even drops down further. The excess fluid and blood are normally removed by the venous and lymphatic systems of the body. The venous system relies on the pumping action of the surrounding muscles to shunt the fluid back to the heart and then to the liver, where it is broken down and redirected. However, because pain and spasm often prevent this muscular action occurring, the fluid will accumulate where the force of gravity dictates.

Elevation, therefore, is an important method of controlling this swelling, with the limb raised above the heart wherever possible. A compression bandage is also desirable.

The application of ice has been shown to have an effect on all these symptoms and is a valuable modality in this phase of rehabilitation.

As discussed earlier, the main use of ice is for its analgesic effects and because ice will not cause fresh bleeding in these early stages. It is the treatment of choice over others which also offer pain and spasm relief.

In these early stages there is also a place for non-heat-producing electromedical modalities such as transcutaneous electrical nerve stimulation (TENS), pulsed ultrasound therapy and various other wave forms, and acupuncture point stimulation.

Applications of heat therapies are not recommended normally in these first 24-48 hours while the damaged circulatory system is healing and unstable and there is a risk of further haemorrhaging.

There is some confusion as to the choice of the modality and its suitability for the task. There is still a great deal of research being undertaken at this moment and the conflicts are many. We would like to elucidate some of the more positive points research has shown in these areas and, compiled with our years of clinical experience, suggest practical guidelines for effective therapy.

However, before discussing pain-relieving modalities, it is necessary to examine the phenomena of pain. As stated previously, the perception of pain is a physiological and psychological process which involves receptors, conductors and integrative cerebral mechanisms. The problem of pain assessment is complicated because it is difficult to differentiate organic from psychic factors and both factors contribute to the final expression of pain.

For many reasons, the patient's perception of pain is not always proportional to the actual structural and functional damage that has occurred, and this may delay the commencement of a positive rehabilitation program. *The immediate aim is to relieve the sensation of pain adequately so that the patient is comfortable, allowing early facilitation of movement.* Above all, it must be remembered that pain is nature's protective device and the use of anaesthetising and pain-block type injections should be administered with the utmost caution and consideration.

There are many ways to modulate pain perception and, in particular, elevate the pain threshold; that is, to afford pain relief. Some of these will be discussed on the following pages.

CRYOTHERAPY

Cryotherapy is the local or systemic application of coldness for therapeutic purposes. The use of cold therapy is ancient, as it was used by Greek physicians to treat acute injuries and, during the Middle Ages, for preparative anaesthesia, as well as on the Russian front during the Napoleonic wars. Because of its long history and general acceptance, a great deal of dogma has surrounded its use and the aims of application are not often understood.

The physiological effects of hypothermia (subnormal body temperature) are many and because of the lack of scientific research in the literature, there are several conflicting aspects which need to be elucidated. However, for the practitioner, several facts are now clear: cryotherapy can be effectively used to treat injury by:

- providing relief of pain in the acute (and indeed later) stage of injury (pain relief);
- reducing secondary hypoxia, oedema and haemorrhage (effect on circulation); and
- providing an effective technique for rehabilitation (cryokinetics).

Pain Relief

This is perhaps the most important effect of ice during rehabilitation. After applying ice to the skin, a sensation of cold is produced, lasting a few minutes. A burning, stinging sensation is then felt and this lasts about five minutes, until a local numbness is achieved. This tends to raise the pain threshold (relieve the sensation of pain). This effect is maintained for as long as the skin temperature is lowered.

As a protective muscular spasm is generally a direct result of pain, the application of ice will also relieve this spasm. Researchers have found that the speed of nerve impulses is governed by the temperature of the surrounding tissues of the receptor site. Cooling has been found to reduce the conductivity of nerves and the effect is proportional to the diameter of the nerve. The reduced conductivity of nerves lessens the sensitivity of the muscle spindle and hypertonicity (spasm) is reduced.

The pain is also relieved by a counter-irritant effect as the cold receptors respond to cooling by a proportionate sharp but transient increase in discharge, and the efferent nerve pathways are bombarded, preventing the sensation of pain reaching the brain.

It is also possible that pain is reduced as the pituitary gland releases endorphins in response to the thermo-regulatory defence mechanisms as the cold invades the tissues. (Endorphins are the body's natural pain inhibitors.)

When aiming to reduce pain and spasm, the optimum temperature appears to be between 12 degrees and 15 degrees C. If aiming to reduce pain only, then 6 to 12 degrees C can be used.

Effect on Circulation

The initial response to cold consists of sympathetic vasoconstriction as the body attempts to conserve heat. This consists of:

1 direct constriction of superficial blood vessels;
2 immediate general vasoconstriction by reflex action through the central nervous system; and
3 delayed general vasoconstriction from activation of the posterior hypothalamus by cool venous blood returning from cooled skin.

Further, this initial vasoconstriction of the injured superficial blood vessels prevents further haemorrhage and a reduction of fluids passing into the tissues, which would produce excessive oedema (swelling).

It has been shown experimentally how the application of ice can control swelling and can limit the magnitude of injury.

Hypothermia reduces the cellular energy needs, thereby reducing the tissue requirements for oxygen; the tissue goes into a state of partial hibernation, minimising the amount of injury. The hypothermia, in fact, causes a marked reduction in metabolic activity and demand of the cooled tissue.

If the tissues in an injured area that escapes destruction by the trauma are not "put into hibernation" by cold applications, their need for oxygen may be greater then the injured vasculature can supply. Consequently, they undergo hypoxic injury. This secondary injury will add cellular debris to the haematoma and increase healing time.

Cold does not appear to reduce the inflammatory response, only delay it. This obviously helps to lessen congestion also in the first 24-48 hours and allows healing to proceed normally.

The literature contains differing reports as to the effect of cold on intramuscular temperature responses. This conflict appears to be due to the variations in severity of the cold treatment, the application time, the site, the surface area over which cold was applied, and the depth at which the temperature was measured.

Many authors have written that cold applications cause an initial vasoconstriction followed by vasodilation and increased blood flow. Some authors claim this effect occurs below 10 degrees C, whereas others suggest 15 degrees C as the turning point.

If the cold application is continued, a sudden deep tissue vasodilation of four to six minutes will occur. This circulatory rush, which is seen as a thermo-regulatory defence against thermal insult, can raise the local temperature sixfold. Vasoconstriction is then re-established, followed by vasodilation in 15-to-30 minute cycles. This cyclic process has been termed "the hunting response".

During continued immersion of the extremities (hands and feet), researchers found that the general level of the peaks of vasodilation often tends to decline, but if the patient is kept warm, alternation of dilation and constriction may occur for several hours.

However, recent research has shown that it is not as simple as that. It appears that cold-induced vasodilation is a very complex mechanism that occurs in different degrees in various parts of the body. It apparently occurs most readily in those areas of the body that are most prone to frostbite, that is, the fingers, toes, cheeks and ears. However, cold packs chilled to -7 degrees C do not present conditions severe enough to elicit vasodilation of the ankle, but some workers have demonstrated a mild vasodilation in the forearm without prior constriction.

Clinically, the benefit of this supposed "hunting response" was to flush debris and exudates from the local area of trauma and enhance healing. Because of the continued conflicting evidence, it is not clear that this positive therapeutic benefit is achieved. On the other hand, because of the other desirable effects of prolonged cold application in these early stages, it will not act in a negative fashion and indeed, may do some good.

A Viable Technique for Rehabilitation—Cryokinetics

The distinction between cold application for acute injuries and cold application for rehabilitation is an important one. After about 48 hours (when the initial acute reaction has settled down), cold may be applied chiefly for its analgesic effect, which then allows early mobility of the injured area. This can be an effective means of rehabilitation, as a 20-minute superficial application of an ice pack produces relaxation, analgesia and relieves muscle spasms. Thus, heat can be effectively produced at a deeper level by active movement which stimulates healing, plus obviously improving local flexibility and strength.

Caution must be used, however, if the patient is asked to exercise vigorously after 60-85 minutes of ice immersion. This immersion has the effect of lowering deep muscular temperature as much as 15 degrees C. Collagen is one of the most important structural materials in the body and is found in abundance in tissues where strength is required; thus tendons, ligaments, muscles and particularly scar tissue are high in collagen content. Cold has the effect of increasing the stiffness of collagen by decreasing its elastic properties. (On the other hand, heat has the effect of increasing tissue extensibility.)

Further, muscle cooling below 20 degrees C delays twitch time and tension during muscle contraction. Cold reduces the discharge rates from the muscle spindle's spiral and flower spray-type ending and also from the golgi tendon organs. Neuromuscular transmission at the end plate is decreased at temperatures below 15 degrees C and totally blocked at 5 degrees C.

Therefore, vigorous stretching techniques may be inefficient or even dangerous after intense icing. Similarly, muscles and tendons may lose some of their protective contractile ability if ballistic stretching or jumping techniques are employed.

Note: Cold therapy should not be used on patients who are unconscious, semi-conscious, have collagen diseases or vasoplastic conditions. An ice reaction (ice burn) can be expected in 15/1,000 cases.

ACUPUNCTURE POINT STIMULATION

The earliest writings on acupuncture go back 4,500 years to its origins in ancient China. "The Yellow Emperor's Classic of Internal Medicine" lays the foundation of Chinese medical thought. It took over 1,500 years to complete, and includes sections on acupuncture, diet, manipulation and massage, hydrotherapy, herbalism, sun and air therapy and exercise.

The important clue from this is that acupuncture was never intended as an holistic approach to medicine as some practitioners would claim now. Its effectiveness would rely on a balance of administration of other medications and recommendations as well.

The traditional theory behind acupuncture is based on the philosophical concept of yin and yang. The Chinese believed the "energy" or a "life force" flows through the body in both a positive and negative aspect and the human organism is regarded as just another manifestation of this energy.

Disease causes an imbalance in this basic energy form and the early Chinese believed that by applying needles at particular points, it is possible to balance the life forces again.

It is doubtful whether these traditional concepts are believed by many medical scientists today, even in China. There has been a great deal of scientific research in recent years into the effects of acupuncture and the possible mechanisms of these effects. Some of the important conclusions can be summarised as:

- Acupuncture has been shown to have various effects on a number of body systems, essentially remedial and analgesic effects.
- Only analgesic effects have been substantiated by scientifically controlled studies.
- The mechanisms of acupuncture analgesia, although not completely elucidated as yet, appear to be a combination of the gate control mechanism as theorised by Melzack and Wall in 1965, and humoral control with enkephalins working through a feed-back loop.
- Stimulation of muscle motor points of the appropriate segmental level, at acupuncture-like frequencies, has been shown to result in the relief of chronic pain.
- Digital pressure, electrical and laser stimulation can be as effective as needling to produce pain relief.
- Where acupuncture point stimulation did have an effect in relieving pain in musculoskeletal conditions, it was considered better results would be obtained by incorporating acupuncture

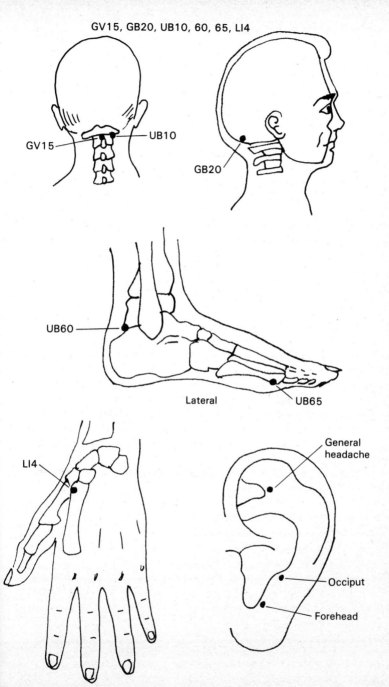

Figure 5.1 Acupuncture point stimulation for headaches, general and occipital.

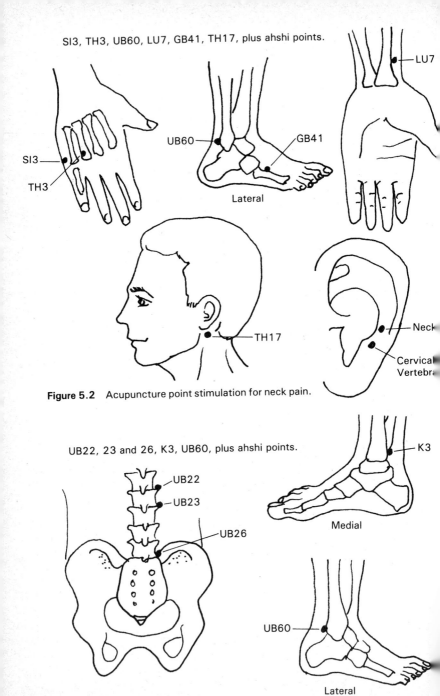

SI3, TH3, UB60, LU7, GB41, TH17, plus ahshi points.

LU7

UB60

GB41

SI3

TH3

Lateral

TH17

Neck

Cervical
Vertebra

Figure 5.2 Acupuncture point stimulation for neck pain.

UB22, 23 and 26, K3, UB60, plus ahshi points.

K3

UB22

UB23

UB26

Medial

UB60

Lateral

Figure 5.3 Acupuncture point stimulation for low back pain.

GB30, 34 and 39, GV 3 and 4, plus ahshi points.

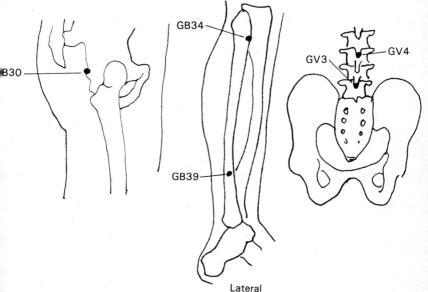

Figure 5.4 Acupuncture point stimulation for sciatica pain.

ST35 and 36, GB34, GV3, plus ahshi points.

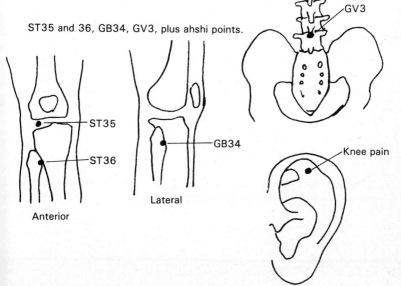

Figure 5.5 Acupuncture point stimulation for knee pain.

BL57, plus ahshi points — *strong stimulation.*

K3, plus ahshi points — *strong stimulation.*

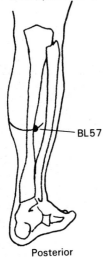

BL57

Posterior

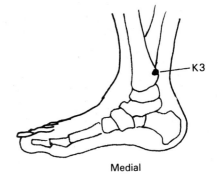

K3

Medial

Figure 5.7 Acupuncture point stimulation for heel pain.

Figure 5.6 Acupuncture point stimulation for Achilles tendon pain.

ST41, GB39, UB60, plus ahshi points.

Ankle

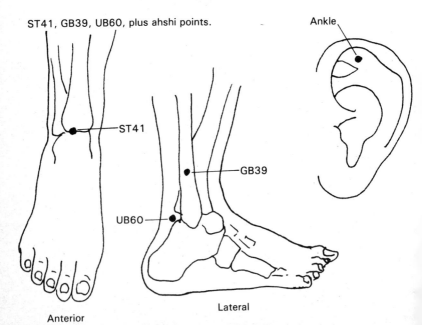

ST41

GB39

UB60

Anterior

Lateral

Figure 5.8 Acupuncture point stimulation for ankle pain.

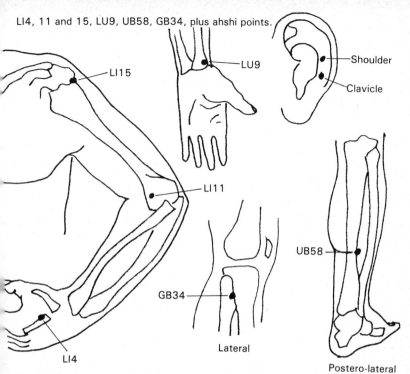

LI4, 11 and 15, LU9, UB58, GB34, plus ahshi points.

Figure 5.9 Acupuncture point stimulation for shoulder pain.

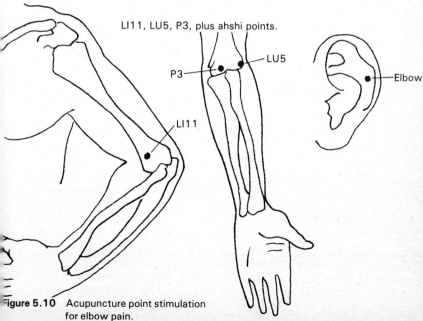

LI11, LU5, P3, plus ahshi points.

Figure 5.10 Acupuncture point stimulation for elbow pain.

LU7 and 9, LI5, TH4 and 5,
plus ahshi points.

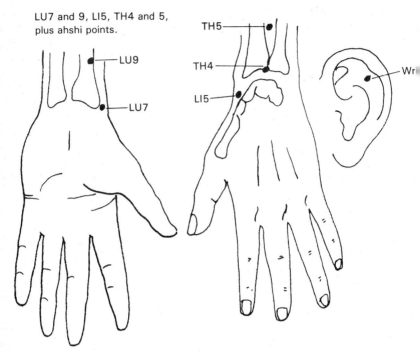

Figure 5.11   Acupuncture point stimulation for wrist pain.

with other modalities and treatment regimes, aiming at a total
restoration of function, not purely at pain relief.

Relief of Pain

It has been found that pain can be relieved by stimulating certain
documented points on the body. In this section, the various body
areas have been dealt with from the viewpoint of pain relief.

For the sake of consistent nomenclature, the points were
referred to by their classical traditional names. The points chosen
have been derived from modern and ancient Chinese sources;
however, some are a result of the authors' clinical experience.
There are doubtless other reflex points which, when stimulated,
are useful in the treatment of pain; however, the following
suggestions have been proven safe and effective.

- If possible, choose a local and distal point.
- Always stimulate the painful area (*ah shi* point), but do not
  use heavy pressure over an acute traumatic injury. Instead,

use ice or TENS (see the section on TENS later in this chapter).
- The effect can be assisted by stimulating the auricular (ear) point.
- Use similar points on the opposite side of body if the effect is not enough.
- When stimulating by digital massage, simply move the fingers or thumbs in rotatory action. To be successful in achieving pain relief, this should induce the desired feeling of heaviness, fullness and tingling that is a forerunner of the anaesthetic effect.

TRANSCUTANEOUS ELECTRICAL NERVE STIMULATION (TENS)

TENS is well recognised for its effectiveness in pain relief. There are many stimulators, electrode types and designs that must be identified and evaluated for workmanship, internal components, engineering and reliability. A standard unit which has been shown

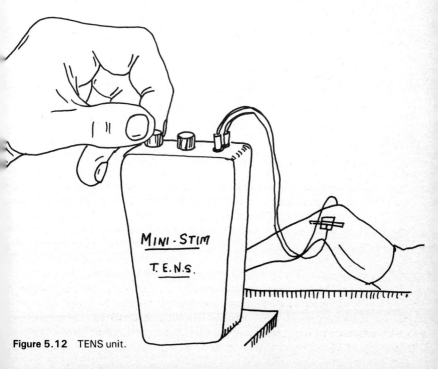

Figure 5.12   TENS unit.

to be effective will have these minimum specifications; a range of output from 0-100 MA, a range of pulse rate from 10-170 pps, and a range of pulse width from 0-600 MU sec.

Effects of TENS

- It modifies the impulses in the sensory pathways.
- It produces a vibrating sensation which alters pain perception.
- The ascending and descending portion of the pulsed current depolarises nerve endings.

Indications for Use

- Effective in modulating chronic, intractable pain syndromes.
- Acute soft tissue pain, particularly in the region of the lower back and the cervical spine and joint and muscle damage caused by sports injuries.
- Arthritic pain.
- Relieving muscle spasm caused by pain.

Contraindications

- Occasional adverse reaction of the skin to the electricity, tape or the conducting medium between the electrode and the skin, particularly if the stimulator is used all, day. Wash the skin and the electrodes regularly.
- Cardiac pacemaker. TENS can be used on the leg but not in the thorax area.
- Do not use over the carotid sinus (neck).
- Pregnancy — not over the abdominal region.

Electrode Placement

Location of the electrodes can be a critical factor in the effective use of TENS therapy. In order to find the best electrode location, placements may be tried at:
- Acupuncture, motor or trigger points.
- The area of greatest tenderness or pain (*ah shi* points for acupuncture).
- Specific dermatomes or spinal segmental levels.
- Distant or contralateral sites.
- Superficial points along peripheral nerves.

Multiple electrodes applied to diffuse areas or to specific anatomical sites and in a parallel or crossed manner may also prove beneficial. A knowledge of anatomy and neuroanatomy is essential to afford the best possible results.

Method of Use

1 Place electrodes in any of the previously mentioned systems or combinations. It may take time, trial and error to find what suits an individual patient.
2 Turn on the machine until the patient feels tingling; the patient then changes the pulse frequency for the most comfortable feeling. He or she may need to increase the intensity as the body adapts to the sensation.
3 If the setting produces pain relief, the patient should feel this after about 20 minutes.
4 Use for about one hour, four times a day, having at least one hour's rest between treatments.
5 Use as little as possible (the patient tends to accommodate if it is left on for too long).

Clinical Experience

The authors have found that the effect of pain relief can be enhanced if the TENS is applied in conjunction with ice therapy. This is particularly the case for acute soft tissue injuries and back and neck conditions which are in a state of severe muscle spasm as a result of intense pain.

Simply apply the electrodes to the painful area or local acupuncture points and place the ice over the electrodes. This then adds the extra beneficial effects of ice.

HEAT AND OTHER ELECTROTHERAPY MODALITIES

When choosing an electrotherapy modality for a particular purpose, the therapist is confronted with a bewildering array of commercial hardware that differs tremendously in effect, performance and price. Individually, they are often marketed as ctrealls and regularly backed by dubious endorsements and suspect research. Overall, the buyer should be aware exactly of what physiological effects to look for from the machine and should be familiar with the relevant research concerning these effects if it is desired to purchase value for money.

It is not intended to review all the electromedical and heating devices on the market. The selection and application of these modalities must be left to the qualified physiotherapist.

Non-heating electrotherapeutic modalities include: interferential currents, galvanic stimulation, pulsed electromagnetic energy, TENS and low dose pulsed ultrasound. In general, all of these devices afford some measure of pain relief, reduce muscle spasm, help control the inflammatory process, help reduce swelling and in some forms enhance the healing process. The precise descriptions of the devices and their physiological responses are left to the appropriate physiotherapy textbooks.

A heating effect can be produced from many sources. Infrared, ultraviolet radiation, hot water bottles, massage and showers or baths are methods of heating the external tissues. Shortwave and microwave diathermy plus continuous ultrasound applications emit an energy form which creates heat within the deeper tissues of the body, such as the muscles, tendons and ligaments. Dosages and administration of these complex devices must be left to the trained therapist.

The important therapeutic effects resulting from heat application are listed here.

Relief of Pain

It is found that a mild degree of heating is effective in relieving pain, presumably as a result of a sedative effect on the sensory nerves. It is most likely that this effect works through a mechanism similar to the application of ice and TENS.

Muscle Spasm Relaxation

By virtue of relieving pain, associated muscle spasm and tension are also relieved. Muscles relax most readily when the tissues are warm.

Increased Extensibility

Heating the tissues results in increased muscle and ligament extensibility which enhances easier stretching and facilitates muscle contractility.

Increased Blood Supply and Metabolism

The application of heat results in dilation of the capillaries and arterioles in the immediately heated area, thus increasing the flow of blood. An increased supply of oxygen and foodstuffs is therefore made available and waste products are removed. This increase in metabolism is greatest in the region where most heat is produced, resulting in an increase in the speed of the healing process.

When choosing priorities, however, it has been shown that muscular work or exercise can increase the heat production ten or twenty times more than the heat production at rest. Exercise after injury, therefore, is important as a means of accelerating metabolism and, in this regard, it is more efficient than applied heat. In view of this, it is recommended that the adminstration of heat should be mainly for its analgesic effect and the subsequent relaxation of muscle spasm.

REGAINING ALL COMPONENTS OF FITNESS OF THE INJURED STRUCTURE

After the acute (or immediate) reaction to injury is controlled, as discussed earlier, in chapter 3, rehabilitative exercises should be commenced to regain all components of fitness of the injured structure.

As mentioned in chapter 2 in "Factors affecting wound healing", prolonged rest and immobilisation can delay early recovery. Because of the inferior quality of the resultant healing scar tissue, it is essential to begin appropriate exercises and activity to remodel and strengthen the new collagenous fibres. *The implications for the sportsperson are considerable if this fact is not recognised.* These factors were further discussed at length in chapter 2.

The specific aims for rehabilitation at this stage are to regain flexibility, strength, endurance, power, co-ordination and skills leading to the normal function of the injured structure.

FLEXIBILITY

It is important to regain flexibility, not only of the damaged structures, but also of the muscles and ligaments around the damaged area. Studies have shown that the best way permanently to lengthen and regain flexibility of connective tissue structures without compromising their structural integrity is by using prolonged, slow intensity stretching at elevated tissue temperatures, and cooling the tissue before releasing the tension.

When a tissue is stretched, it may exhibit elastic or plastic properties or a combination of both. Elastic stretch represents a spring-like behaviour where the effect of the stretch is temporary or recoverable. Plastic stretch infers that the tissue *retains* its new shape after the elongated stress is released. This is permanent elongation and is the desirable end product when dealing with scar tissue.

Temperature has a significant influence on the mechanical behaviour of tissues under tensile stress. Heating increases extensibility and recent studies have demonstrated that, at about 44 degrees C with a given amount of stretching, a greater proportion of plastic deformation will occur. Cooling the tissues before releasing the tension apparently allows the collagenous microstructure to restabilise more toward its new stretched length.

As stated previously (chapter 1, "Prevention of Injury in Sport"), slow, static stretching techniques should be the method of choice as these procedures will override the protective stretch reflex and allow the muscle and any other damaged structures to increase in length.

A contract-relax technique is used with best effect. The muscle needing to be stretched or the muscle controlling the joint or structure needing to be stretched is resisted strongly in the opposite direction of the stretch for 6 seconds. The patient then relaxes and a strong controlled sustained stretch is applied in the opposite direction for 10 seconds. The patient is allowed 20 seconds for recovery and the process is repeated twice more.

To increase the chance of permanent plastic effects occurring, ice should then be applied for about 20 minutes with the structure in a sustained stretch.

STRENGTH

As discussed earlier in chapter 2 ("Factors affecting wound healing"), it was seen how scar tissue is never as strong as the tissue it replaces. For rehabilitative purposes, strength should be considered in three sub-categories: strength, power and muscular endurance. Depending on the particular sport and the individual's specific needs, the program will be aimed at overloading one or more of these parameters.

Strength is the maximum force that can be exerted in a single, all-out effort. A weightlifter aims for this type of strength.

Muscular endurance is the ability of a muscle to contract repeatedly or to sustain a contraction against continued resistance.

Long distance runners, rowers, mountain climbers and crosscountry skiers will need to redevelop this type of muscular fitness.

Power implies explosive action or the ability of a muscle to exert force with speed. High jumpers, boxers and shotputters need to develop power to excel at their sports.

To compensate for this lack of strength in the scar tissue, it is important for the sportsperson to participate in an intensive, well-planned strengthening program. Where the injury has occurred in a musculotendinous unit (such as a hamstring muscle), he or she must undergo a retraining program to develop strength, power and endurance of the unit (depending on the sport played). Similarly, for an injured joint structure, the athlete must strengthen the muscles controlling the joint as the joint tissues will strengthen as the muscular workload increases.

Where movement is restricted at any stage of rehabilitation (because of pain, swelling, spasm or plaster), isometric contractions serve the purpose until a progressive resistance program of isotonic or isokinetic contractions can be instituted.

An isometric exercise is one in which no joint movement occurs and the contraction is against a fixed resistance, for example the other hand, doorway or wall. Each contraction should be applied with maximal pressure for a minimum of six seconds.

An isotonic exercise is one where there is a change in muscle length as a resistance is moved through a range of movement (for example a barbell, weight, boot or brick).

Isokinetics is a method of exercise at controlled speed and accommodating resistance. The muscle is made to work at its maximum capacity throughout its whole range of movement. It incorporates the factors of work, power, force and endurance available through both isotonic and isometric exercises. The only drawback with this form of exercise is that it requires expensive, specialised equipment.

It is clear, both from clinical observation and from experimental evidence, that a tissue is only as strong as the function placed on it. So, if you consider that a chain is only as strong as its weakest link, and the weak link is obviously the healing scar tissue, it is essential to design and implement a specific and general retraining program.

CO-ORDINATION

When soft tissue is injured, nerve endings and nerve pathways are inevitably damaged and when a joint capsule is damaged in any joint injury, a certain amount of reflex arc, that is, the sequence of nerves involved in a reflex action, is lost. This leads to a lack of motor co-ordination, a tendency for joints to give way and for slowed reflexes when performing specific or general movements. It is therefore important to include co-ordination exercises in the rehabilitation program. For instance, a cricketer with a damaged shoulder may need to undergo such a program incorporating the myotatic reflex for bowling. (When a muscle is stretched out fully, it initiates the myotatic reflex which produces a stronger and faster contraction.)

Similarly, a footballer after an ankle injury will need to regain motor co-ordination and proprioception. (Proprioception is the sum response to a great many different "stimuli" sent to the brain or spinal cord by nerve endings in muscles and joints). For players it mainly means balance and joint position sense.

REGAINING FUNCTIONAL ACTIVITY

As stated at the beginning of this chapter, rehabilitation begins immediately after injury and continues until the patient is ready to return to his or her sport. Athletes must be restored to *full* competitive fitness at the earliest possible moment. It is important to recognise that an athlete has a much higher level of cardiovascular fitness, that is fitness of the heart and lungs, than the untrained individual. Athletes must, therefore, appreciate the urgency of dynamic early therapy to maintain this fitness. The importance of the "treat and train" attitude has been effectively shown in studies of bed rest and training. When untrained subjects were rested for a 20-day period, it took them only 10 days to regain their maximal oxygen intake (which is a measure of their cardiovascular fitness), but it took trained athletes up to 40 days to regain their previous fitness level.

Never let athletes be idle because of injury. The rest of the body should still be made to work strongly; swimming, running, punching, weight training or whatever they are capable of doing. Furthermore, they must begin retraining for their sport as soon as possible while they are still receiving treatment for their specific injury. In other words, an athlete with a hamstring injury must start jogging, within limits of pain, as soon as possible. Likewise, a tennis player with a "tennis elbow" must start replaying tennis at pain-free levels, while the elbow condition is still being treated.

The point is, the damaged area must be retrained specifically through all the skills of the proposed sport so it may functionally adapt to the stresses of that sport.

All of these factors reinforce the need for the institution of an early, active, positively directed rehabilitation program based on the need of the individual athlete.

PART III
SPECIFIC INJURIES

This part has been written mainly for the clinician who is consulted by sporting patients. Of course the layperson with an interest in sports first aid and the coach should derive benefit from the information that follows, as they can be involved both in the rehabilitation program and certainly in the application of the methods of prevention that are suggested. It is extremely important for the aware sports first aider to understand the mechanisms of the various injuries discussed and be able to institute proper preventative measures as part of the training and coaching program.

The injuries have not been selected entirely arbitrarily. Experience has shown that these particular injuries occur more commonly than others among people who play sport.

Each injury is discussed in a similar, methodical way. The incidence and mechanism of the injury are explained, together with a brief description of any functional anatomy that may be involved. The management of the immediate treatment of the injury is then presented, followed by a more detailed discussion of the principles and methods of treatment of the later stages of the injury. Important points for the progression of the treatment plan leading to full functional rehabilitation are noted. Finally, methods to prevent the injury recurring are also considered.

Of necessity, some injuries are dealt with in more detail than others, particularly the most consistently occurring ones, notably the ankle, knee and shoulder injuries. The proper management of these injuries should be under the daily supervision of a physiotherapist experienced in the special interest of sports medicine. There can be no substitute for experience based on a sound knowledge of anatomy, wound healing, exercise physiology, treatment techniques and progression, electrotherapy modalities, and injury prevention. Coaches and first aiders, therefore, should work with the club doctor and physiotherapist as a team for the benefit of the player in the prevention and treatment of injury.

6
UPPER LIMB INJURIES

The most common injuries to the upper limb in body contact sport occur to the shoulder girdle and finger (metacarpal joints). Overuse injuries occur also at the elbow and wrist joints, as well as the shoulder.

The three types of injuries which are dealt with in this chapter are outlined here.

Shoulder Girdle Injuries

- acromioclavicular joint;
- sternoclavicular joint;
- glenohumeral joint dislocation;
- rotator cuff impingement syndrome.

Elbow Joint Injuries

- "tennis" and "golf" elbows (medial and lateral epicondyle overuse syndromes)

Wrist and Hand Injuries

- wrist ligament sprain;
- fractured scaphoid;
- PIP (proximal inter-phalanges) and DIP (distal inter-phalanges) joint strains of the finger;

SHOULDER GIRDLE INJURIES

The glenohumeral joint is a modified ball-and-socket joint which allows for a great range of movement around the shoulder. This great mobility has a tradeoff in sport, particularly contact sport, as stability is often compromised. Because of the long levers involved and the many intricate and heavy actions required, the joints of the shoulder girdle (fig. 6.1) are often damaged.

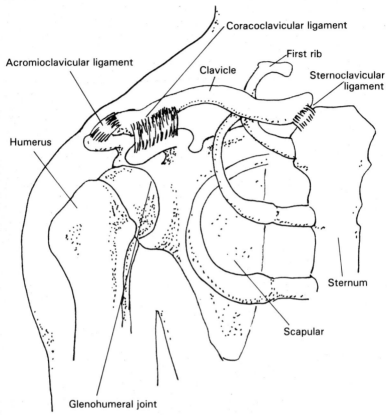

Figure 6.1 The joints of the shoulder girdle.

ACROMIOCLAVICULAR JOINT

The acromioclavicular joint is a relatively unstable joint which is often damaged during contact sports. Injury typically occurs when the point of the shoulder is speared into the ground or into an opposing player or post. It can also be caused by a direct kick or a fall on the outstretched hand. Depending on the extent of injury, it generally results in a swelling on top of the shoulder, with pain on touching this point, and a limitation in the range of shoulder movement (grade 1 injury). A grade 2 sprain will display damage to the coracoclavicular ligament as well and the clavicle will be raised slightly in relation to the acromial process.

A grade 3 sprain indicates complete rupture of both the acromioclavicular and coracoclavicular ligaments, and results in very obvious elevation of the clavicle. This injury is particularly prevalent in rugby players, obviously because of the tackling inherent in the game.

Early Treatment

Regardless of the extent of damage, pain relief and prevention of excessive swelling are the two most important aims. Ice packs, analgesics and a compression pad over the joint must be applied. The shoulder and arm should be supported, either with a sling or taping, to prevent further damage as the weight of the arm may stretch the injured ligaments further.

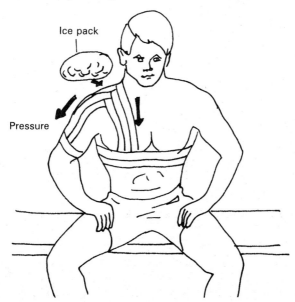

Figure 6.2 Strapping and ice for an acromioclavicular joint injury.

Late Treatment

It is rare for the ligaments to be so extensively damaged that reconstruction or reparative surgery is necessary. Most of these injuries can be managed satisfactorily by a conservative treatment program. For an occasional grade 3 sprain, particularly with concomitant injuries, and considering cosmetic results (for example, the prominence of the distal clavicle compared to a surgical scar), surgery may be the treatment of choice. Other factors such as age, demands of a particular sport, time and money involved with surgery, plus normal surgical risks should also be considered. In fact, all types of treatment may finally result in a normal pain-free, functional shoulder, the main difference being time.

In the early stages, pain will dictate the amount of movement possible, so an isometric exercise regime must be instituted to maintain muscle tone (fig. 6.3).

Assisted range of motion exercises should then be introduced, progressing to non-assisted or isotonic exercises, always within the limits of pain (figs 6.4 and 6.5). As the flexibility improves, resistance should be correctly applied to gain strength, endurance and power of the muscles controlling the joint.

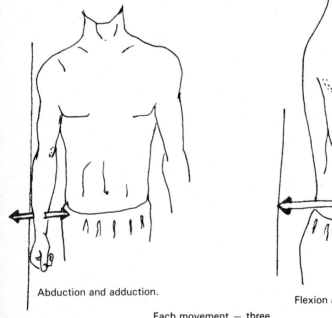

Abduction and adduction.

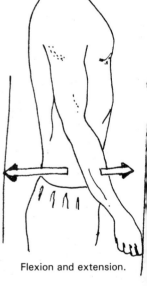

Flexion and extension.

Each movement — three six-second holds.

Figure 6.3 Isometric exercises.

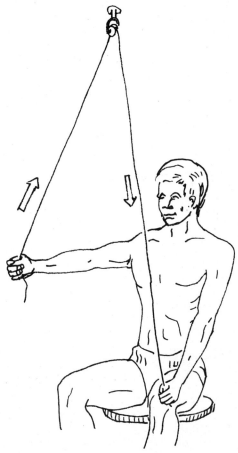

Figure 6.4 Assisted exercises — flexion, extension and abduction movements.

When executing exercises in the standing position it is important to work both shoulders at the same time. This stabilises the trunk, so "trick movements" or "compensation movements" don't fool you into thinking the shoulder joint is moving, when in fact other joints are moving to compensate for the loss of shoulder mobility, either because of pain, spasm, adhesions or calcification.

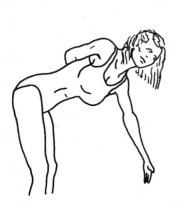

a. Pendulum exercises; back and forward, side to side and rotation.

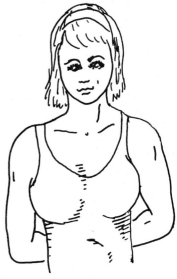

b. Internal rotation, moving to c.

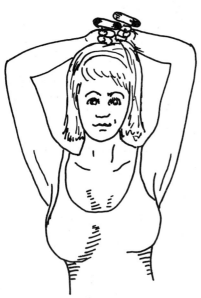

c. External rotation.

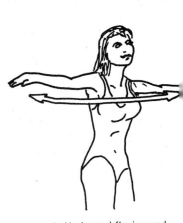

d. Horizontal flexion and extension.

Figure 6.5 Isotonic exercises. As the range of joint movement improves, resistance or weights should be commenced for all exercises. To increase strength, use progressively heavier weights.

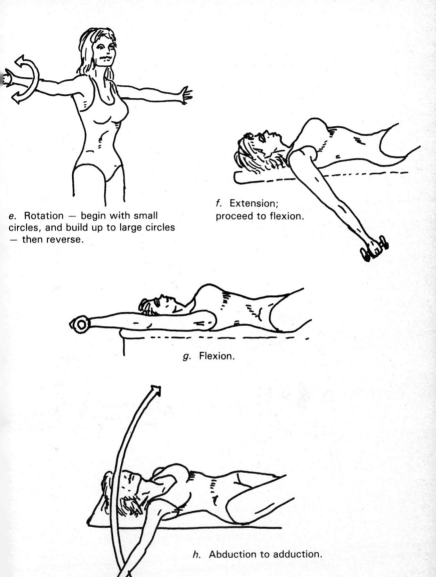

e. Rotation — begin with small circles, and build up to large circles — then reverse.

f. Extension; proceed to flexion.

g. Flexion.

h. Abduction to adduction.

Figure 6.5 Isotonic exercises (continued).

Prevention

It is virtually impossible to strap the acromioclavicular joint satisfactorily to prevent it from being damaged. If it needs to be strapped, the player probably shouldn't be playing as he or she hasn't built up enough strength in the injured area. Often adhesive plaster over the joint will give a particular person a great deal of confidence, yet it can be of little physical value.

Good padding in shoulder pads *should* prevent this injury, as in theory it softens and distributes the blow. It is doubtful, however, if many shoulder pads on the market today serve this purpose. Care must be taken also to prevent the padding from being so strong that it can be used as a weapon.

Finally, the best prevention of this injury must be a successful strength, endurance and power training program, aimed at increasing the energy-absorbing qualities of the ligament involved.

STERNOCLAVICULAR JOINT

The sternoclavicular joint (fig. 6.1) is not damaged often in sport as little movement takes place in and around the joint. It anchors the clavicle onto the sternum and as the clavicle is a stabiliser for the shoulder joint proper, it is mainly injured by violence to this joint or by telescopic action from a fall or tackle on the outstretched arm (fig. 6.6).

The grade 1 sprain is characterised by tenderness and swelling around the joint, with little disability or loss of shoulder function. The grade 2 sprain, however, will limit shoulder abduction and be painful on horizontal flexion as the clavicle is approximated to the sternum. There will be mild subluxation and more obvious distortion and swelling. The treatment for both grades 1 and 2 sprains is immediate ice therapy, followed eventually by heat and an exercise routine exactly the same as in figures 6.3, 6.4 and 6.5 for shoulder rehabilitation.

A grade 3 sprain may be more serious, as there is gross ligament damage plus joint separation.

If the clavicle is displaced posteriorly, it may apply pressure to blood vessels and/or the trachea which may interfere with breathing. The bone should be reduced by a physician and the joint immobilised for at least a week (fig. 6.6). When pain and swelling permit movement, rehabilitation exercises should be commenced as for the shoulder routine.

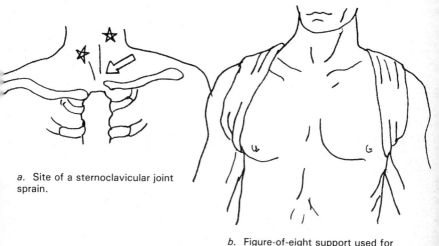

a. Site of a sternoclavicular joint sprain.

b. Figure-of-eight support used for immobilisation of the sternoclavicular joint.

Figure 6.6   Sternoclavicular joint sprain.

GLENOHUMERAL JOINT DISLOCATION

The most common of all shoulder joint dislocations is the anterior dislocation of the glenohumeral joint. It occurs generally as a result of violent contact, either with another player or an obstacle such as the ground or goal post. The arm is forced into abduction and externally rotated. An excessive throwing action may also dislocate this joint.

The damage may be quite extensive as the greater tuberosity of the humerus is pushed out of its labrum, perhaps damaging it on the way, plus stretching or tearing the glenohumeral ligament, the anterior joint capsule and possibly the rotator cuff muscles as well. Fractures may occur to the glenoid or to the greater tuberosity (the end of the humerus) and additional common complications may arise from damage to the brachial nerve and axillary artery.

This injury is accompanied by intense pain and an immediate protective muscle spasm of the shoulder girdle muscles. There will be an obvious indentation where the deltoid muscle should be as the humeral head slides forward and the patient will strongly resist

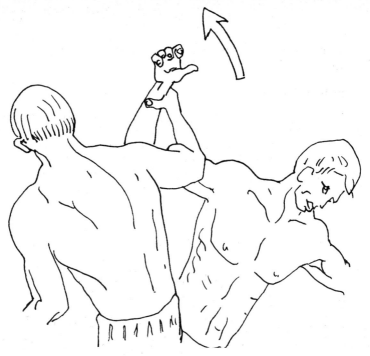

Figure 6.7 Typical mechanism of an anterior glenohumeral joint dislocation.

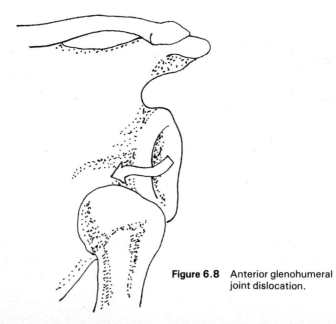

Figure 6.8 Anterior glenohumeral joint dislocation.

arm movement across the chest (that is, adduction and internal rotation).

Immediate Treatment

This injury requires immediate reduction, preferably by a physician or well qualified physiotherapist.

The shoulder should be first packed in ice as soon as possible to control the pain and relieve the spasm. There are several effective reduction methods in use. The two which the authors use with good effect are the Hippocratic method and the Stimson method.

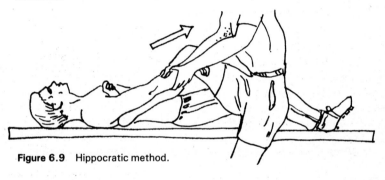

Figure 6.9   Hippocratic method.

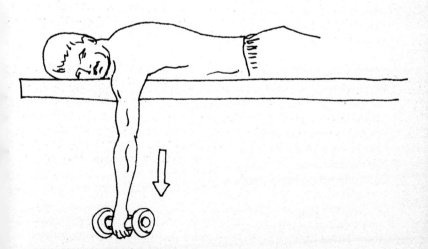

Figure 6.10   Stimson method.

The Hippocratic method therapist is shown in figure 6.9. The therapist places a bare foot in the axilla, being careful of nerves and vessels. Apply *gentle* traction.

The Stimson method is shown in figure 6.10. The patient lies supine on a table with the dislocated arm hanging over the edge. A weight increases the traction to accomplish reduction.

Because the Hippocratic method incorporates a risk of damaging blood vessels and nerves, the Stimson has less chance of incurring complications. If these methods fail, the patient must be transported to hospital immediately to be manipulated under anaesthesia.

After reduction, the shoulder should be immobilised in a sling in a position of internal rotation.

Late Treatment

There is considerable controversy as to the duration of immobilisation as various authorities suggest anywhere from one week to four weeks. If there is no fracture, we recommend that exercise should be commenced as soon as possible within limits of pain. This, of course, will vary with the intensity of damage.

Isometric exercises, however, can be commenced within two or three days and, as soon as pain permits, pendulum exercises can be added, as in figure 6.5. As flexibility and strength improve, movement can be progress to the routine suggested in figure 6.5. However, care must be taken, once abduction to 90 degrees is reached, to respect external rotation movements, as the joint is most vulnerable in this position.

Recurrent Shoulder Dislocation

No matter what conservative treatment has been instituted early, it has been found that a great number of glenohumeral joint dislocations will recur. This is because if there has been significant damage to the shoulder capsule and glenohumeral ligaments so as to create an unstable joint, no amount of rest (immobilisation) or exercise will alter this status. Further, the extent of damage is rarely obvious on initial consultation and treatment. While a specific, vigorous exercise rehabilitation program may dynamically develop sufficient stability with some injuries, it is obviously not a panacea. We contend that if a shoulder dislocates three times after a positive exercise therapy program has been undertaken, the athlete should consider a surgical procedure; there are several efficient options available.

Repeated dislocations will occur with progressively less force each time and will continue to stretch the supporting structures, leading eventually to damage to the cartilaginous structures of the joint itself (arthritis). Above all, a trick shoulder which dislocates readily is a potential threat to life; for instance, the shoulder may "give" when hopping onto a train.

Recurrent Subluxation of the Shoulder

This condition is more obvious in the repetitive actions of the throwing sports or swimming, particularly backstroke. It implies a partial dislocation of the humeral head, where joint continuity is transiently lost during the subluxation. There is a feeling of insecurity when the shoulder is externally rotated whilst in abduction. This is a positive "apprehension sign" test. The patient complains of vague shoulder pains and a feeling of instability after bowling or executing certain movements.

A differential diagnosis must include an X-ray to rule out a chip fracture of the antero-inferior rim of the glenoid. If this is negative, treatment must be aimed at improving the integrity of the soft tissue structures supporting the joint. Once again, a positive exercise program developing the flexibility, strength, power, endurance, proprioception and function of all shoulder muscles, tendons, ligaments and capsule must be carried out.

If this routine doesn't adequately treat the condition, the patient must consider surgical intervention similar to the anterior dislocation procedures.

ROTATOR-CUFF IMPINGEMENT SYNDROME

This condition is discussed in detail in part IV, chapter 10.

ELBOW JOINT INJURIES

The most common injuries to the elbow joint are to the medial and lateral epicondyles. The main cause is overuse. These injuries are discussed in detail in part IV, chapter 10.

WRIST AND HAND INJURIES

WRIST SPRAIN

Because of the intricate and versatile movements which the wrist allows and the delicacy of the bones and supporting structures which form it, the wrist is often damaged in sport. The most common cause is from a fall on the extended or hyperextended

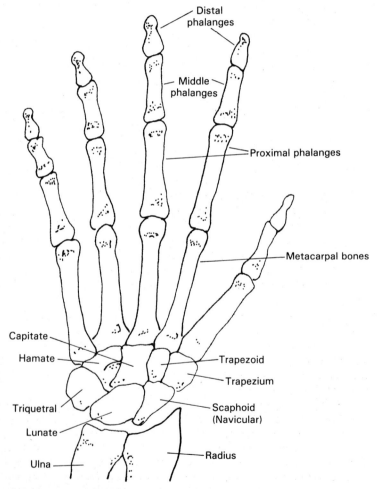

Figure 6.11 Bones of the wrist.

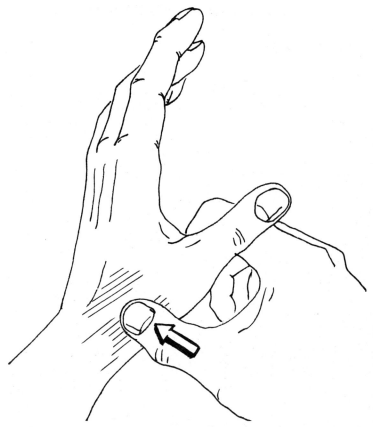

Figure 6.12 Palpation of the scaphoid bone through the anatomical snuffbox.

wrist. However, excessive jarring from power movements in racquet sports can also overload this joint. The most common injury is a ligament sprain to either the anterior or posterior ligaments supporting the wrist.

Any athlete with a history of a fall should be routinely X-rayed to determine possible fractures, the distal radius (Colles' fracture) and the scaphoid being the two most common fracture sites. It is important to keep in mind that a fractured scaphoid does not always show up on a normal X-ray immediately and it may take some weeks until it becomes evident radiographically. If there is suspicion of an undisclosed fractured scaphoid, a nuclear bone scan may be needed to ascertain an earlier more accurate diagnosis.

A sprained wrist will have generalised swelling, point tenderness and limitation of wrist movement, whereas a fractured scaphoid will have virtually no swelling, reasonable joint movement and pain on compression of the scaphoid bone.

It is, of course, highly likely that both injuries will occur with the same accident, so it is vital to secure a positive diagnosis, as the fractured scaphoid *must* be immobilised to aid healing and prevent possible complications of mal-union and non-union.

The treatment for a localised ligament strain is along classical lines; ice, compression and elevation for the first two days, then exercises to regain range of joint movement, muscular strength, power and endurance plus normal function. A dynamometer (wrist grip tester) is a useful tool to gauge initial strength and then to assess improvement at various stages (fig. 6.13).

Exercises for the wrist are shown in figure 6.14.

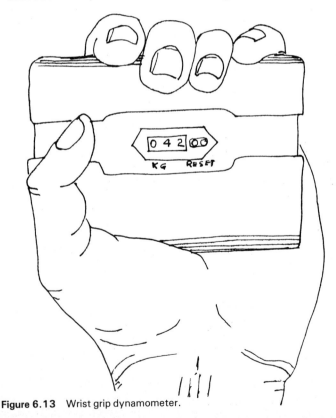

Figure 6.13   Wrist grip dynamometer.

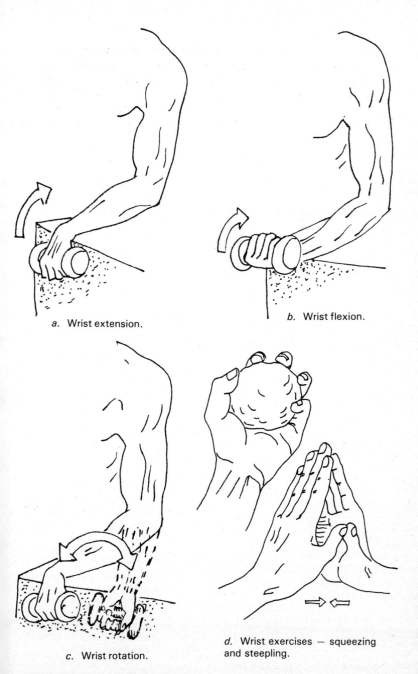

a. Wrist extension.

b. Wrist flexion.

c. Wrist rotation.

d. Wrist exercises — squeezing and steepling.

Figure 6.14   Exercises for the wrist.

Taping

Procedure 1

Mild injury. This technique will give reasonable support, but still allow a functional range of joint movement. Use a 2 cm elastic adhesive bandage and, incorporating a spica for the thumb, finish with a spiral on the forearm (fig. 6.15(a)).

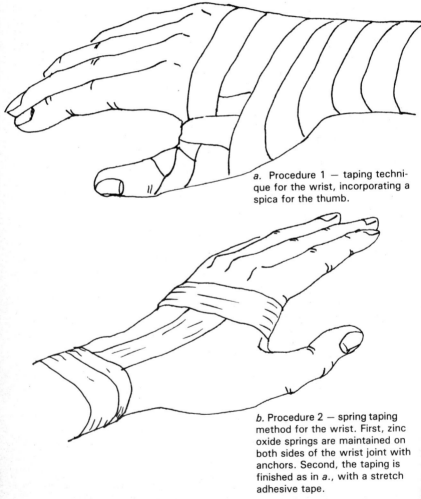

a. Procedure 1 — taping technique for the wrist, incorporating a spica for the thumb.

b. Procedure 2 — spring taping method for the wrist. First, zinc oxide springs are maintained on both sides of the wrist joint with anchors. Second, the taping is finished as in *a.*, with a stretch adhesive tape.

Figure 6.15   Taping for the wrist.

Procedure 2

More severe injury. Spring technique. This procedure maintains the wrist reasonably secure at about 15 degrees extension, the position of function. The spring allows small movement. Use a 2 cm zinc oxide tape for the anchor and spring and finish with 2 cm adhesive plaster as in procedure 1 (fig. 6.15 (b)).

INJURIES TO THE HAND, FINGERS AND THUMB

The most common injuries to this region are dislocations, sprains and fractures of the phalanges. All three types of injuries occur

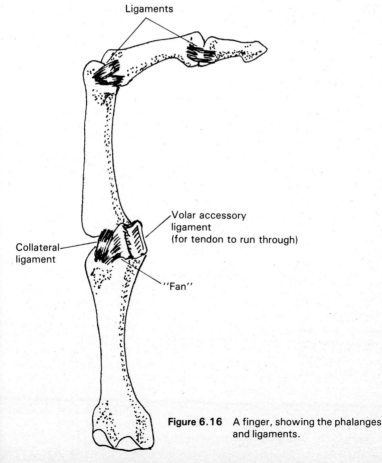

Figure 6.16 A finger, showing the phalanges and ligaments.

from a similar mechanism; external force from a fall, blow or twisting action.

The obvious signs of fractures are deformity, crepitus and excessive movement. If these signs are not present and a fracture is suspected because of localised tenderness over the shaft and only a little swelling, an X-ray is necessary. Treatment is mainly by immobilisation by splinting, depending on the extent of damage; always refer to a physician.

A dislocation of the finger involves mainly damage to the capsular tissue, but because of the extent of damage and the possibility of a small fracture, these injuries should be X-rayed also. There is considerable scarring from this injury and the joint must be mobilised as soon as pain permits. Passive mobilising techniques are very important, as well as resisted exercises to regain normal function and to prevent "lumpy" swollen phalanx joints.

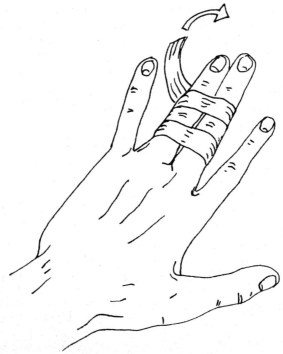

Figure 6.17   Taping of phalanges, allowing mobility.

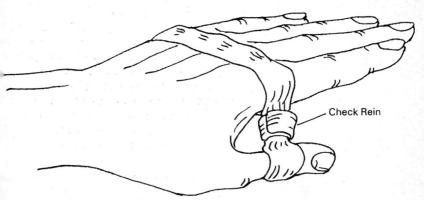

Check Rein

Figure 6.18   Spring taping method for the thumb.

The same procedure is necessary for sprains of phalanges. As with any ligament and capsular damage, pain, swelling and limitation of movement are the early obvious symptoms. The digit should be packed in ice to help control these symptoms, then an exercise rehabilitation program should be instituted.

Once again, the aim is to prevent excessive scarring from limiting movement and strength, so full range-of-movement exercises should be persevered with, both passive and active.

For a severe sprain, splint it to the digit beside it for support. As mobility improves, tape as figure 6.17 to allow more normal function.

7
LOWER LIMB INJURIES

Common injuries to the lower limb can be conveniently classified into two main headings: muscular injuries and joint injuries, as shown here.

Muscular Injuries

- haematoma (contusion, cork or charley horse);
- quadriceps strain;
- hamstring strain;
- groin pain; (a) adductor muscle strain, or
  (b) osteitis pubis;
- gastrocnemius strain (calf muscle).

Joint Injuries

- knee;
- ankle.

MUSCULAR INJURIES

Muscles are injured either by a direct method, such as an external blow or force, perhaps from an opponent's shoulder, or indirectly, either from a sudden powerful muscular contraction resulting in the tearing of muscle fibres, or alternatively, from continual repetitive stress from exercise causing microtrauma to either a muscle or the musculotendinous unit.

HAEMATOMA

All muscle injuries, no matter what the cause, generally result in a haematoma. However, in sports medicine, a "haematoma" classically refers to an injury caused by direct violence. A haematoma may also be known as a "contusion", "cork" or "charley horse". It results from a blow or some external violence to a

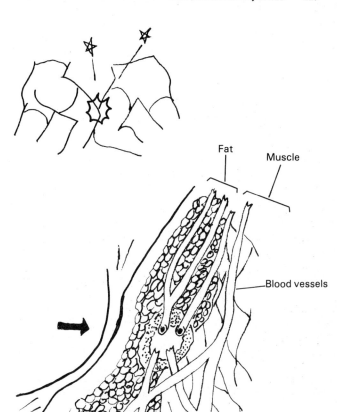

Figure 7.1 Blow on the thigh causing a haematoma. Blood, fibrin and cellular fluid seep into the tissues, causing swelling, pain and loss of function.

muscle, typically an opponent's knee hitting the player's quadriceps, the large muscle group on the front of the thigh. This violence causes damage primarily to blood vessels, resulting in blood seeping into the surrounding tissues. There is generally only minor damage to the muscle tissue itself, although obviously the full extent of the injury will depend on the force of the blow and the state of preparedness of the injured muscle (whether relaxed or contracted) during the impact; the stronger the contraction, the less severe the damage.

Another factor which can determine the amount of bleeding

can relate to the amount of blood in the area at the time of impact. The more strenuous the effort, the more blood could be expected to be pumped to the muscle to aid performance. This may lead to either intramuscular or intermuscular bleeding or both. Because it is not possible to diagnose the extent of damage accurately for up to 72 hours, conservative treatment must be instituted immediately otherwise the complications from this injury can be extremely incapacitating.

Diagnosis

Players will generally know if they have been hit, although occasionally, in the heat of the moment, with adrenaline pumping, minor knocks aren't always noticed. There will be pain, either at rest or on movement with palpation, and there will often be associated protective muscle spasm. There will generally be swelling within a few hours and, depending on the extent of the injury, bruising (ecchymosis) may track down the thigh and even into the knee or further into the calf. There will be loss of quadriceps function and, because the quadriceps normally supports the knee joint, the knee may even be painful and tend to give way.

The injured athlete will have trouble contracting (tightening) the muscle and there will be pain on bending the knee, that is, stretching the thigh muscle. A significant, deep haematoma which is neglected may later harden and calcify, forming heterotopic bone formation, commonly called *myositis ossificans*. This hard, egg-shaped mass in the muscle bulk will form if the injury is pushed too hard in the early stages, preventing full mobility of the limb. In rare cases, surgery may be needed to remove this calcification but mostly, after a six-week rest period, the muscle will return to full function with the following treatment program as for a normal haematoma.

Immediate Treatment

The important aims in the early stages of treatment are to relieve pain and muscle spasm and to prevent and reduce excessive bleeding and swelling. The application of ice and a compression bandage with the foot elevated should be continued until swelling has been controlled. Thus, as soon as the player leaves the field, pack moist, crushed ice on the thigh for up to 30 minutes; this should be repeated three or four times for the day and, possibly, the next day as well.

As there is not normally a great deal of damage to the muscle tissue itself as in an intermuscular type injury, gentle stretching exercises can be started on about the second or third day. *Warning:* at this stage, the exercises are only intended to relieve muscle spasm and pain, so never push past the point of pain; if too much tension is placed on a deep intramuscular injury, complications may arise.

Massage

In our opinion, there is no place for massage in this early stage as inexperienced probing fingers might increase the bleeding of the torn blood vessels. Massage has a wringing effect and there may be a place for it after a few days as practised by an experienced masseur to help break down the hardened clots. Massage also has a heating and therefore an analgesic and relaxing effect. However, the use of massage in this instance should never be overplayed and should never replace the use of active exercises in the rehabilitative process.

Late Treatment

The important aims of late treatment are to regain full muscle extensibility, strength, power and endurance and to regain full function specifically related to the patient's sport.

Exercises should be commenced after application of some heating modality to aid extensibility and muscle contractibility.

Because of the natural weakness in the healing scar tissue of the damaged area and because of the role of the quadriceps in maintaining knee stability, it is important to begin a gradual progressive overload resistance program as soon as pain and swelling permit. Such exercises as straight leg raising and knee extension over the edge of a bed (see figs 7.2 and 7.3) will contract the quadriceps. Passive exercises to regain flexibility should be continued, such as the patient grasping his or her own ankle from behind (with a rope, perhaps) and bending the knee so that the ankle touches the buttocks, within limits of pain, of course. The athlete should continue building up to a full squat stretch until the buttocks rest on the heels, then leaning back as far as possible (fig. 7.4).

As strength and flexibility improve, the aim is to regain power and endurance by working out on isokinetic variable resistance equipment (such as Cybex, Hydragym, and so on).

As soon as the player can walk normally, encourage jogging,

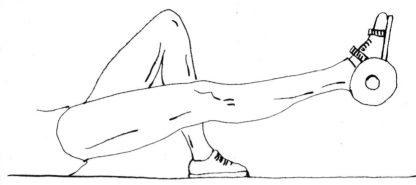

Figure 7.2 Straight leg raises. Lift the leg about 30 cm, hold, and then lower. The opposite knee may be bent to take pressure off the back.

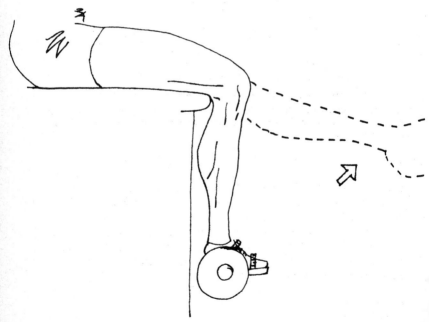

Figure 7.3 Knee extension.

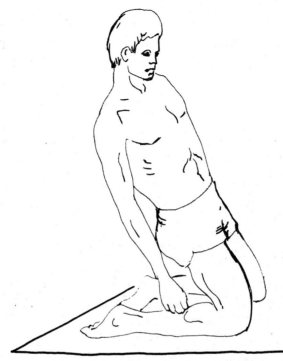

Figure 7.4   Deep squat stretch. The athlete should build up gradually to a full squat stretch; the buttocks rest on the heels, and the athlete leans back as far as possible.

gradually working up to running at full pace, then introduce specific skills related to the patient's chosen sport. This functional retraining program should be carried out concurrently as flexibility and the other fitness components improve.

Be prepared to treat each patient and injury individually, understanding that the severity of the injury in respect of pain, swelling and movement loss will dictate the progress from the acute phase to the later stage.

Prevention

It is, of course, impossible to prevent collision occurring in body contact sports. Fitness and consequent alertness and agility may be a help, but the only real support can come from an intensive weight training program to gain muscular strength, durability and resilience.

QUADRICEPS STRAIN

The quadriceps is the large muscle group on the front of the thigh. It comprises four muscles and runs over two joints, the hip and the knee. Collectively, the muscles work to flex the hip and extend the knee and together with the reciprocal action of the hamstring group, they enable normal locomotion to take place.

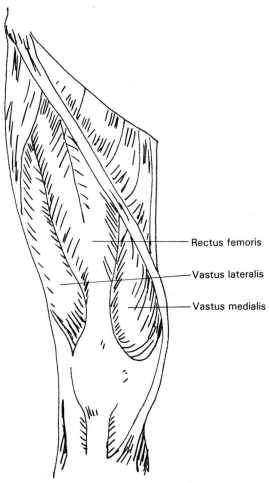

Rectus femoris

Vastus lateralis

Vastus medialis

Figure 7.5 The quadriceps muscle group; a fourth muscle, the vastus intermedius, is situated under the other three.

The most common site of injury or strain is in the rectus femoris, the long muscle running over the hip joint which lifts the thigh up as in running. Very rarely do any of the lower three muscles sustain a strain, although it does certainly occur. Collectively, these three muscles straighten the knee and particular importance is placed on the large vastus medialis, or "dewdrop" muscle, on the inside of the thigh above the knee. This muscle extends the knee the last 15 degrees, enabling the joint to "screw home" and thus straighten the knee for walking. Its other prime function is to align the patella in its groove on the femur to prevent the patella (kneecap) tracking incorrectly and causing patellofemoral pain (see chapter 9).

Mechanism of Injury

This injury generally occurs when athletes suddenly accelerate, particularly if they have not had a sufficient warm-up or when they are getting tired towards the end of the game and try to sprint for the line. Muscle imbalance in right and left limbs has been suggested as a predisposing factor in these strains, as has an inadequate quadriceps/hamstring strength and power ratio.

Diagnosis

The patient generally feels the muscle "go" and will complain of pain anywhere from below the hip bone prominence down the muscle to just above the knee. The muscle is generally painful on palpation, particularly over the musculotendinous junction of the rectus femoris muscle itself. Athletes may experience pain on stretching the muscle (as in a squat) and on contracting the muscle (as in a straight leg raise). A severe strain will exhibit swelling, spasm and eventually ecchymosis (bruising).

Early Treatment

As soon as the player leaves the field, moist crushed ice should be packed on the thigh for half an hour; this should be repeated about three times a day for at least 24 to 36 hours. This will help to ease pain and muscle spasm and control swelling and bleeding. A crepe bandage may give support to the thigh as well as help to control the swelling.

Late Treatment

As with other muscle injuries, the important aim is to prevent

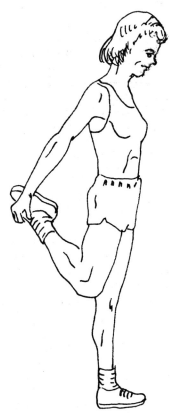

Figure 7.6 Standing stretch.

the healing scar tissue from limiting normal movement, so stretching exercises should be started within limits of pain. A deep squat stretch (fig. 7.4) and a standing stretch (fig. 7.6) are the two most effective exercises to achieve this.

Second, an overload weight training course should be started to ensure the injured unit regains adequate strength and endurance. Straight leg raising (fig. 7.2), knee extension (fig. 7.3) and hip flexion (fig. 7.7) are important exercises. Another is long hip flexion with the knee bent (fig. 7.8) as this simulates the running action.

At the same time, isokinetic-type training programs should be commenced to retrain the power component of muscle fitness.

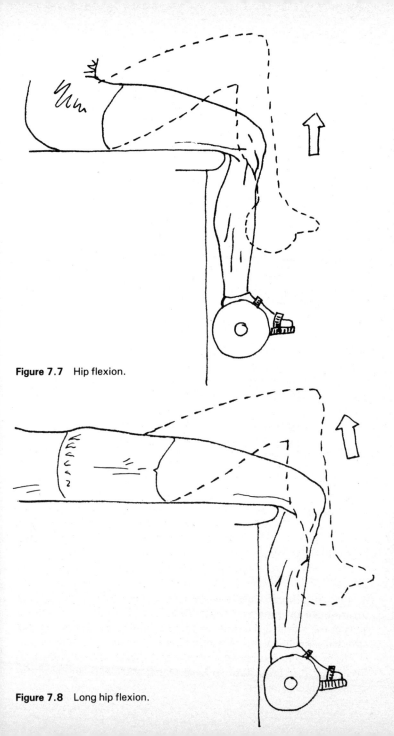

Figure 7.7 Hip flexion.

Figure 7.8 Long hip flexion.

Finally, the injured person should begin functional training as soon as possible by running at whatever speed he or she can manage, up to the point of pain. However, experience has shown that athletes should not resume their sport for at least a week after they have reached top speed. This extra time appears to be needed to build the necessary functional endurance to last a full game through.

Prevention

An adequate warm-up before training and playing is essential. (See "The warm-up",chapter 1.) As well, a properly co-ordinated fitness training program should be followed, with particular attention given to resistance training (weights and isokinetics) and training relating to the individual sport.

HAMSTRING STRAIN

The hamstring injury is one of the most common problems hindering athletes. Inadequately treated, it can be one of the most debilitating and confidence-breaking hurdles to a sporting career. The injury is most often experienced by the speed athletes of the sporting world, the track athletes and the back line of a rugby team.

The hamstrings are the large group of muscles on the back of the thigh, originating from the large bone in the buttock (seat bone), running down the back of the leg where two of the muscles attach below the knee on the inside and the other attaches on the outer aspect of the knee (fig. 7.9)

Mechanism of Injury

Several reasons have been suggested as predisposing factors in hamstring strains.

Inadequate Warm-up

It is essential that the player stretches the muscle to its fullest before both training and competing. This should be one of the aims of the warm-up; that is, to gain full flexibility of the muscles, otherwise the injury may occur in the first few minutes of the game or the first few metres of a sprint race because of inadequate flexibility. It is important to keep warm and flexible during the game also, as on a cold day the muscles may tighten again,

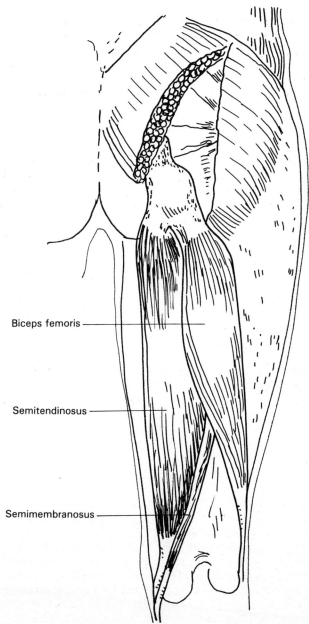

Biceps femoris

Semitendinosus

Semimembranosus

Figure 7.9 The hamstring group of muscles.

particularly during a rest break or during a quiet period of the game.

Inadequate Fitness

Another group of hamstring strains will occur at the end of a race or game when extra strength, power and endurance may be called for. Other fitness parameters such as flexibility and co-ordination must also be adequate. Stress is often placed on the muscle when a running player bends down to scoop up the ball on the ground. Because the hamstring runs over two joints (the hip and knee), and the muscle is on full stretch while the player is bending, the extra strain required to contract (or shorten) the muscle while stretching can often overload it and cause damage. This may be related to the fact that the biceps femoris receives two separate nerve supplies, one to the long head and one to the short head. This may have the effect of confusing the co-ordinating skills of the muscle group as one part of the muscle is relaxed and the other contracted. It is important, therefore, that a properly co-ordinated overload training program be instituted to achieve full functional fitness in all parameters (see chapter 1).

Muscle Imbalance

Another reason for hamstring injuries may be a muscle imbalance in the strength/power ratio between the quadriceps muscle group on the front of the thigh and the hamstrings. Whereas various ratios have been suggested, it is more likely the correct ratio for an individual may be specific to the demands put on the athlete by the sport in which he or she competes. Therefore, a co-ordinated isotonic and isokinetic resistance training program should be carried out on both groups, otherwise there will be an unevenness in speed of muscle contraction and a muscle strain may result.

Muscle asymmetry in right and left limbs has been suggested as another reason for muscle strains, so this fact must be considered in the co-ordinated program.

Other factors which have been attributed to hamstring strain, either singularly or in combination, include fatigue, poor posture, poor form, improper skill patterns, magnesium imbalance, anatomic variations and abnormal muscle contraction.

Diagnosis

The hamstring injury is extremely easy to diagnose. The patient generally feels something "go" or "snap" at the back of the thigh. It is often preceded by a small muscular "spasm" or "twinge" before the snap, but this awareness is rarely registered by the patient as a warning of a strain. A strain is characterised by pain, tenderness, protective muscle spasm and swelling at the site of injury. Bruising (ecchymosis) may appear at practically any section of the hamstring muscles. In fact, after a few days, the force of gravity may cause the bruising to track into the knee, the back of the calf, or even into the ankle area. The track athlete generally injures his or her leg at either end of the hamstring mass, but the footballer generally injures the hamstring in the lower third of the muscle belly. There is pain on both active contraction and passive stretching.

If there is no history of trauma in the muscle itself and the onset of thigh pain is gradual and doesn't appear till the day after the event, low back damage with sciatic nerve involvement must be suspected. A thorough vertebral column assessment must be undertaken to eliminate fascial, ligamentous or discogenic pathology.

It is possible to confuse a mild grade 1 hamstring strain with the early incipient "spasm". Note that a strain will be made worse on stretching, but a "spasm" will be relieved by stretching. This, of course, can dictate treatment considerably. Finally, most hamstring strains are grade 2, or moderate. A grade 3 strain, which constitutes a rupture, is rare, as is the prospect of surgery. All grades generally react well to conservative therapy.

Early "Spasm"

Treatment

If this minor twinge is detected before a strain occurs, the best treatment is application of ice or ultrasound plus a slow stretching technique. This appears to relieve the spasm within 24 hours and as long as a balanced exercise program is instituted, the patient should not miss a game. The cause of this spasm is generally unknown.

Muscle Strain

Early Treatment

As the muscle is rarely completely ruptured, there will be a partial tear of one of the muscles or at one of the musculotendinous junctions. Athletes should never continue to play on with a hamstring strain and they should be retired from the game. The damaged muscle should be packed in crushed, moist ice for at least half an hour every three or four waking hours for the next 36 to 48 hours. A compression bandage can help prevent and control excessive swelling. The important aims in this period are to relieve pain and reduce muscle spasm, plus limit swelling and bleeding.

Late Treatment

Once pain and muscle spasm have been relieved and the swelling has been controlled, the aims of treatment are to regain all fitness parameters. Specifically, this will generally mean to stretch the healing scar tissue to strengthen it (including improving power and endurance) and to regain full function. These can all be worked at concurrently so that by the time the hamstring has regained full flexibility and strength, the athlete should be running at top speed.

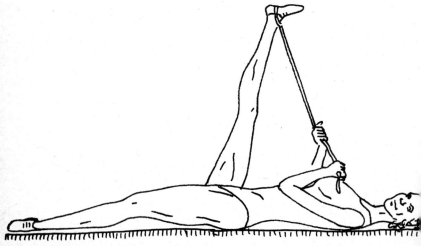

Figure 7.10 Hamstring stretch.

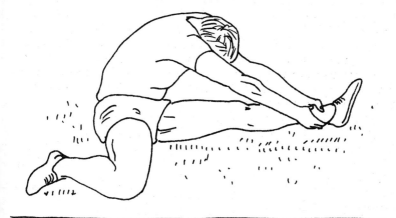

Figure 7.11   Hurdler's exercise.

Stretching   Stretching exercises are begun as soon as pain permits. The patient ties a rope around his or her foot and passively stretches the leg to the limit of pain (fig. 7.10). The leg is held in this position for about ten seconds; it is then relaxed for about twenty seconds, then stretched again, repeating this cycle about five times. Each stretch should slowly extend further into the range. This effect will be enhanced if the leg is warm before you commence the stretching routine, so the application of a heat modality before stretching is worthwhile. A progression is then to add the hurdler's stretch using the static stretch technique (fig. 7.11).

A slow, static stretching technique is more desirable than ballistic or sudden forced stretches which may cause more damage if executed too vigorously in the early stages. Other stretching exercises such as touching toes (with straight back), head to knee bends and the stretches shown in chapter 1 (fig. 1.3(d)), all improve muscle length. It is important to do these often, at least two or three times a day, and also to exercise both legs.

Strengthening   When strengthening the hamstring, it is important to remember that it runs over both the knee and the hip joints. It must be placed on full stretch to gain the maximum benefit from the contraction (see the exercise shown in fig. 7.12). To achieve an overload, wear a weight boot and increase resistance as the program dictates. At the same time, an isokinetic training program should be commenced to retrain the power component of the muscle fitness.

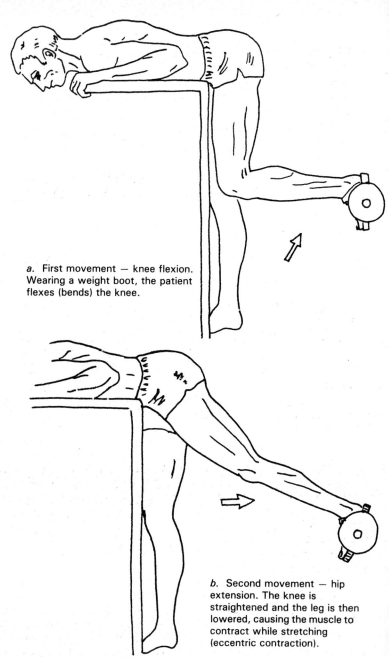

a. First movement — knee flexion. Wearing a weight boot, the patient flexes (bends) the knee.

b. Second movement — hip extension. The knee is straightened and the leg is then lowered, causing the muscle to contract while stretching (eccentric contraction).

Figure 7.12 Hamstring strengthening exercise.

Full Function   While this process is going on, the patient should begin jogging as soon as possible, within limits of pain. Once the patient builds up to a sprint on flat ground, running up stairs and hill climbs help to overload the muscle. Once again, as with the quadriceps muscle strain, it is important not to return to competition too early. It appears that a week of sprinting at full speed is essential to regain functional endurance, otherwise the risk of recurrence is high.

Note: Because of inadequate treatment and the risk of continued recurrence, this injury is often accompanied by apprehension and depression. The only way to overcome this worry is to assess meticulously all fitness components, looking for deficiencies in flexibility, strength, power, endurance or co-ordination, and questioning overload techniques with training, diet and rest and so on. Confidence in the muscle is only regained after inadequacies are identified then fastidiously and patiently tackled.

Prevention

As mentioned previously, a warm-up before training and playing is essential. As well, a properly co-ordinated fitness training program should be followed, with particular attention to resistance training and strong overload running to strengthen the leg adequately.

GROIN PAIN

Many patients present with a condition loosely labelled as "groin pain". The condition occurs most frequently in sprinting sports and ones which require great rotational forces at the hips, such as soccer, hockey, jumping events (long jump particularly) and rugby. The pain may be brought on suddenly by a particular single event or insidiously by continued repetitive movements causing microtrauma over a period of time.

As a variety of structures may be involved or damaged, it is vital a careful examination is carried out. A differential diagnosis must consider the following muscles and their tendons, attachments and associated joints; iliopsoas, rectus femoris, adductor group and the pubic symphysis (fig. 7.13).

The two most common injuries are to the adductor group and the pubic symphysis (osteitis pubis) and these will be discussed in detail.

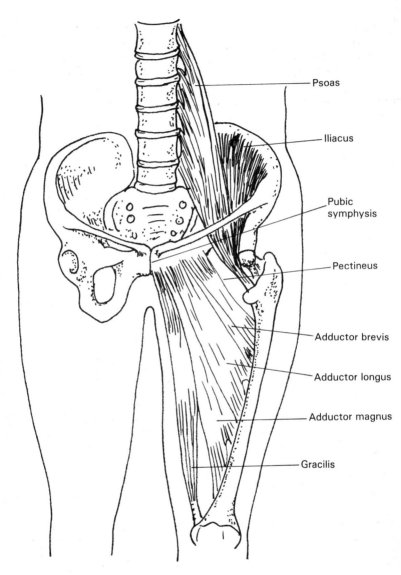

Figure 7.13 The groin — showing major structures.

Adductor Muscle Strain

Damage to the adductor muscle group typically strikes people who have to sprint and are required to change direction suddenly while running, such as soccer and hockey players. As contact sports have become more aggressive and dynamic, injury to this muscle group is now common. The primary action of the adductor muscle group is to drag the leg towards the middle line of the body. For example, it is used when the leg is swung across the body as in striking for a ball and it stabilises the leg on the pelvis while the pelvis and other leg rotate around as in changing direction. Sudden swerving actions, and indeed propping actions in this direction, often overload the muscles and a strain generally occurs in the muscle bulk or to the tendinous attachment of the bone.

The adductor muscle group has the secondary action of assisting the hip while it is flexing and extending, as in lifting the thigh forwards and backwards. Consequently, when great speed is required, the adductor muscle group assists the action which can overload the group and cause damage. This is very much the case with track sprinters and the speed athletes of the sporting world.

Diagnosis

Understanding the biomechanics of this injury is important, so a careful history must be taken, particularly in relation to the player's movements and the pain location. As groin pain may also be referred from various orthopaedic conditions of the hip, sacrum and lower back, a thorough assessment of these areas should be undertaken. Other structures which may give groin pain are the rectus femoris muscle, the sacroiliac joint, the iliopsoas muscle and the pubic symphysis.

To test for adductor group strain, the athlete must sit or lie with knees bent and legs apart (hips fully abducted, that is). He or she is then asked to squeeze the legs together (into adduction), against the operator's resistance. This will cause a painful response if there is an adductor muscle strain.

Early Treatment

The immediate reaction of muscles to pain is to contract in a tight spasm as a protective mechanism to prevent more damage. This primitive reflex can hinder early rehabilitation, so the important immediate aim is to relieve the pain and therefore lessen the consequent spasm. The application of ice for this reason is one of the most essential requirements of early treatment. Furthermore, the ice will help to control bleeding and swelling. A crepe bandage comfortably wrapped around the thigh will help to support the injury.

Late Treatment

After the second or third day, depending on pain and spasm, an exercise routine should be started to prevent the healing tissues

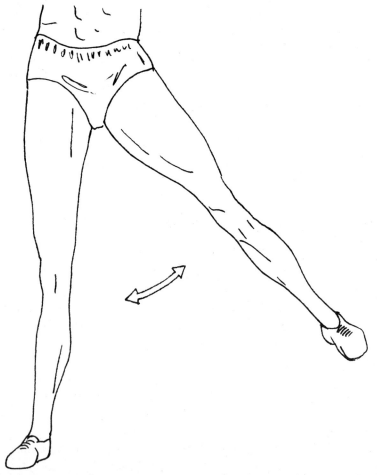

Figure 7.14   Stretching exercises, standing, for adductor muscle strain.

forming a restrictive and weak scar. Before each exercise session begins, some form of heat should be applied to further aid in pain and spasm relief and to increase tissue extensibility.

Stretching Exercises   Stretching exercises are begun by standing on the sound leg and gently swinging the injured leg forwards and backwards (flexion and extension movements), and then across and away from the body (adduction and abduction movements). All movements are to be executed up to the point of pain. It is important to exercise both legs in turn for this routine, as the extra stress of weight bearing introduces an overload component to begin strengthening (fig. 7.14).

To stretch the damaged fibres more specifically, sit on a mat (or table) with knees bent to a position where most pressure will be placed on the injured area when the thighs are pushed apart (abducted). Apply appropriate stretching techniques in this position (fig. 7.15). Other stretches for the adductors and hip muscles were illustrated in chapter 1 (fig. 1.3).

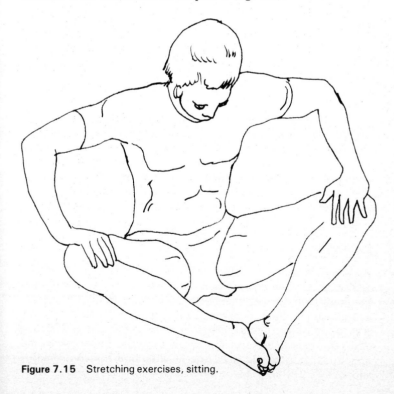

Figure 7.15   Stretching exercises, sitting.

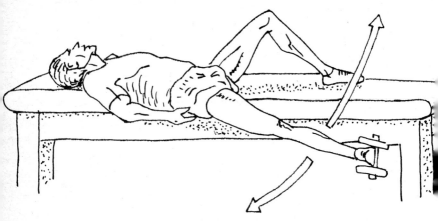

Figure 7.16   Adductor strengthening exercise.

Strengthening Exercises   The most effective technique for strengthening the adductor group of muscles is to use a weighted shoe in a carefully overloaded resistance program, lifting the leg through as full a range of movement as possible (see fig. 7.16). Once again, both legs are exercised in this fashion.

Functional Retraining   It is important to start functional activity as early as possible also during this period. Once athletes can walk without a limp, they should be encouraged to jog, then to improve to quarter pace, to half pace, and eventually to full speed, all within limits of pain, of course. When they can sprint at full pace in a straight line, they should then carefully begin changing pace and direction, running in a circle, zigzags and figures-of-eight, eventually introducing skills appropriate to their particular sport.

It is unwise to compete until a whole week of full activity has been achieved because it takes as long as this to regain functional endurance in the injured muscle.

Prevention

An effective warm-up program is essential before each training session and before competition. However, once again, fitness is the main ingredient in the prevention of this injury. A specific and general training program, both pre-season and during the season, must be undertaken to ensure a flexible and strong adductor muscle group. The thigh muscles, lower back and abdominal muscles all need special attention for co-ordinated support.

Osteitis Pubis

Traumatic osteitis pubis is a stress injury to the symphysis pubis. It is common in soccer players, particularly those participating at a skilled level. Other athletes who seem to be troubled by the condition are track and field competitors in the disciplines of triple jump, broad jump and hurdles, distance runners and rugby players.

Athletes affected with this condition will complain of a combination of the following symptoms:

- an aching pain in the groin radiating down the inside of the leg, sometimes bilaterally;
- lower abdominal pain spreading across the anterior abdominal wall;
- testicular pain which may also be bilateral; sexual function is often hampered.

History

Patients usually experience increasing groin and abdominal pain over many weeks. The pain will eventually become severe during

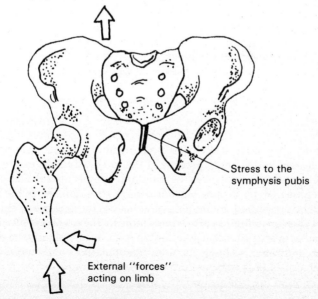

Impingement of the sacroiliac joint

Stress to the symphysis pubis

External ''forces'' acting on limb

Figure 7.17 Mechanism of injury.

or some hours after competition and then gradually subside over the next few days. A common pattern is that the athlete competes on the weekend which induces the pain. The symptoms then gradually subside and by mid-week the athlete can train lightly, and is thus available for the next weekend competition. This pattern continues until sports performance is affected and the pain becomes so severe that assistance is sought.

Mechanism of Injury

An external force applied to the end of the limb produces a shearing stress to the symphysis pubis and often the sacroiliac and lumbar spine joints are involved (fig. 7.17).

In sport, the injury is often a result of overuse, in which microtrauma or repetitive overloading eventually leads to the clinical presentation. In some cases, one traumatic incidence such as a scrum collapse in rugby may precipitate the condition.

Examination

The basis of the examination is to differentiate between traumatic osteitis pubis and an adductor muscle strain. (See table 7.1.)
The lumbar spine, hip joints and sacroiliac joints should also be tested, as a strain of these joints and their associated structures can also be present.

Management — Acute Phase

The only treatment of choice in the acute phase is *rest* from all pain-producing activity.

Symptomatic relief can be administered in the form of ice and electrotherapy modalities such as TENS and ultrasound. All rehabilitative exercises which would be prescribed for an adductor strain (that is, the stretch and strengthening routines) are contra-indicated in this phase because of the tortional forces exerted on the symphysis pubis. As the pain and symptoms subside, light exercises which do not place excessive stress on the pubic area can be prescribed. Swimming obviously is the exercise of choice.

When examination procedures indicate the involvement of the lumbar spine, sacroiliac joint or hip joint, local palliative regimes are indicated. These include manipulative and mobilising techniques plus various forms of electrotherapy.

Table 7.1 Differentiation of traumatic osteitis pubis from an adductor muscle strain.†

Osteitis pubis	Adductor strain
History Usually a slow, progressive increase in symptoms	There is a definite history of trauma producing an acute soft tissue injury.

Site of pain and tenderness

Abdominal pain

Point tenderness

Referred pain to testicle

Acute tenderness at site of injury

Adductor muscle pain

Diffuse adductor pain

Radiology X-rays may show erosion of the symphysis pubis. Nuclear bone scans may display "hot spots" indicative of bony stress.	No radiological change

† Dunn, R.N. — "Traumatic Osteitis Pubis", *The Australian Journal of Physiotherapy*, 1986, vol. 32, no. 1.

Rehabilitative Phase

A "reduced activity" period of approximately four to six weeks is necessary to achieve a pain-free state. The athlete should be reassessed once symptom-free. The common finding is lack of muscle flexibility in the adductors, hip flexors, hamstrings and the erector spinae. A lack of flexibility in these muscle groups is probably a predisposing factor to this injury.

The rehabilitation program should include comprehensive passive stretching and stretching exercises for the tight muscle groups. Isotonic and isokinetic muscle strengthening routines should be given to all muscles stabilising the pelvis, especially the abdominals, hip extensors and back extensors.

A graduated return to sports activity must be carefully monitored and supervised. The recurrence of traumatic osteitis pubis is easily precipitated with a training overload. If the athlete is allowed to return to high training loads too quickly, symptoms will reappear leading to prolonged recovery times.

GASTROCNEMIUS STRAIN (CALF MUSCLE)

The calf muscle incorporates the gastrocnemius muscle, the soleus muscle and the Achilles tendon (fig. 7.18). Damage to any of these structures occurs typically in running and jumping sports, but most injuries are suffered by the thirty-to forty-year-old squash or tennis player.

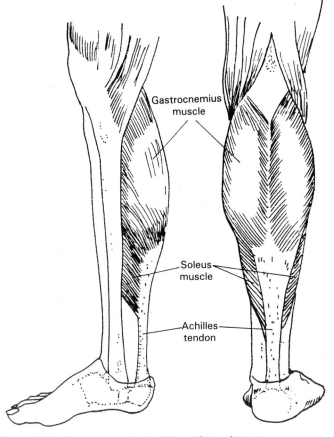

Figure 7.18   Side and rear views of the calf muscle group.

Diagnosis

The player generally feels as if the calf muscle has been hit from behind by another player and hears a loud snap as the muscle fibres tear. The damage usually occurs at the junction of the medial head of the gastrocnemius and the Achilles tendon. The injured player may collapse in pain and can take no further part in the game.

It is important to differentiate between a muscle strain and a complete Achilles tendon rupture. The Achilles tendon's prime function is to plantar flex the foot (allow it to point down). However, even if the tendon is completely torn, it may still be possible for the athlete to perform the function because the other plantar flexor muscles, namely the posterior tibial, peroneal and toe flexor tendons can continue to achieve this action. The Thompson test, therefore, can be a valuable aid in correctly diagnosing this injury (fig. 7.19).

If the gastrocnemius muscle is strained, there will also be pain on palpation, plus local swelling. Eventually, after several days, ecchymosis may track down the course of the leg to the foot, being influenced by the force of gravity.

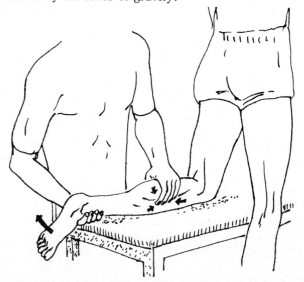

Figure 7.19 The Thompson test. With the patient kneeling, foot extended over the table edge, squeeze the calf just below the widest circumference. If the Achilles tendon has lost continuity, the foot will not plantar flex, and the test is then positive for a ruptured tendon.

The cause of this injury is the same as that of other muscular injuries. The player may not have warmed up enough and ensured a good stretch in the muscle before playing, or may not have been specifically fit to play a hard game.

Early Treatment

Early treatment is aimed at alleviating pain and spasm and controlling excessive swelling so normal principles of ice application, compression and elevation as described in chapter 3, the section on "Immediate treatment of soft tissue injuries", are essential for the first 24 to 48 hours. This injury is greatly influenced by gravity so the leg should be elevated above the level of the heart, on a chair or pillow, and a compression bandage applied. The patient may need crutches or a walking stick for the first few days as bearing weight will certainly inflame the condition.

Late Treatment

As soon as pain permits, exercises should be commenced to regain normal muscle flexibility and then to regain all components of strength and fitness. The aim is to stretch and strengthen the healing scar tissue, building up to normal function.

Stretching Exercises

As the calf muscle runs over two joints, the knee and the ankle, full stretch will only be achieved with the knee straight and the ankle dorsiflexed (bent up). Begin with the knee in flexion, over the edge of a table, and then extend (straighten) the knee. Further, bend the toes and ankle up and back to gain full calf stretch. Hold this for about 10 to 15 seconds, then repeat, always to the point of pain (fig. 7.20).

Strengthening Exercises

These can be commenced as weight-bearing exercises, with the body weight being shared and distributed from one foot to the other as a resistance. Eventually, take the weight fully on the injured leg, raising onto the toes. To increase the effect, stand on a doorstep or a gutter and stretch right down and come right up (stretching and strengthening in one exercise) (fig. 7.21). To isolate the soleus muscle, the knee of the affected leg must be bent to relax the gastrocnemius muscle, allowing the soleus to then be

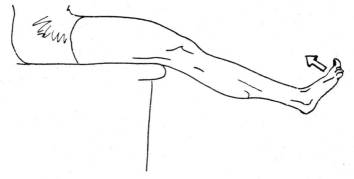

Figure 7.20 Stretching exercises — non-weight-bearing.

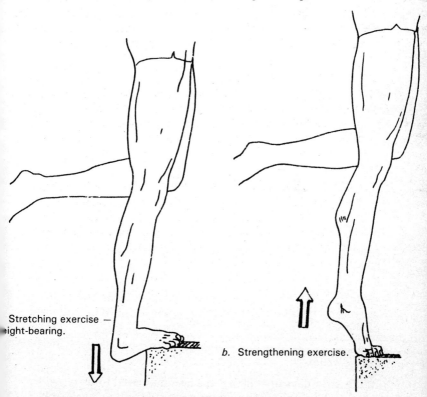

Stretching exercise — weight-bearing.

b. Strengthening exercise.

Figure 7.21 Stretching and strengthening the calf muscle.

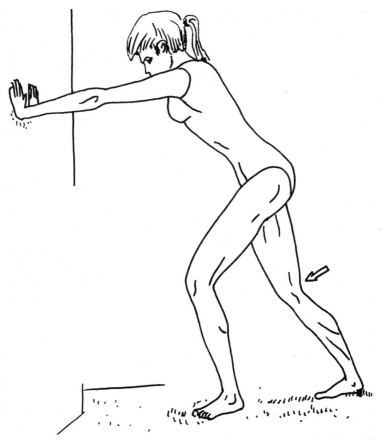

Figure 7.22 Stretching exercise for isolating the soleus muscle — bend the knee.

stretched (fig. 7.22). At the same time, an isokinetic training program should be commenced to regain the power component of the muscle fitness.

Full Function

In the early days of walking, the heel may need to be raised by a heel cushion pad to stop overstretching of the torn muscle (place a 1 cm felt pad under the heel inside the shoe) (fig. 7.23).

As soon as patients can walk without a limp, they should be

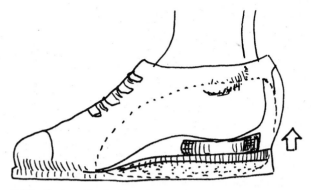

Figure 7.23   Heel cushion inside a shoe.

encouraged to jog and then to build up speed to their normal functional level. Once they can run at full speed, they should train at this standard for a week before they compete again as it appears to take as long as this to develop functional endurance in the muscle.

Prevention

Once again, the patient should get fit to play sport, not play sport to get fit. The need for this may be reflected in the number of middle-aged achievers who sustain this injury. They are generally of a competitive nature and rely on their mental toughness to win. However, they need more. A proper conditioning program, including specific strengthening and flexibility exercises for the calf muscle group, should be planned and followed. The program should also be sports-specific, including at least three runs a week and possibly two or three squash or tennis sessions a week.

As well, a comprehensive warm-up should be mandatory before every training and playing session. For the calf, 10 to 20 slow, deep stretches should be undertaken in addition to the normal program.

JOINT INJURIES

KNEE INJURIES

The knee joint is a complex yet stable modified hinge joint, well developed by evolution to function very efficiently in normal circumstances. Unlike other mammals (except elephants), humans have the distinction of bearing weight upon this joint in extension, instead of in the flexed position which acts as a shock absorber for other species. This fact renders the joint very vulnerable as the stresses placed upon it by extreme athletic pursuits make the incidence of knee injury very high among people playing sport.

Functional Anatomy

To be able to localise a particular condition, it will be necessary to revise certain aspects of the functional anatomy of the knee.

The knee is not a simple hinge joint. It is bicondylar and this allows the tibia to rotate in its longitudinal axis to various degrees of knee flexion with maximal rotation occurring at 90 degrees flexed position. No rotation occurs in full extension (fig. 7.24).

Knee locked while in extension

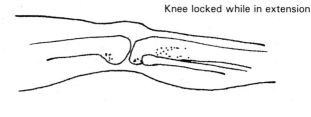

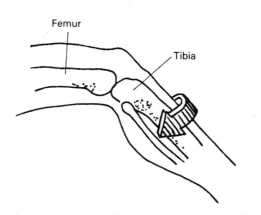

Tibia rotates on the femur as the knee bends

Figure 7.24   Showing tibia rotating as the knee bends.

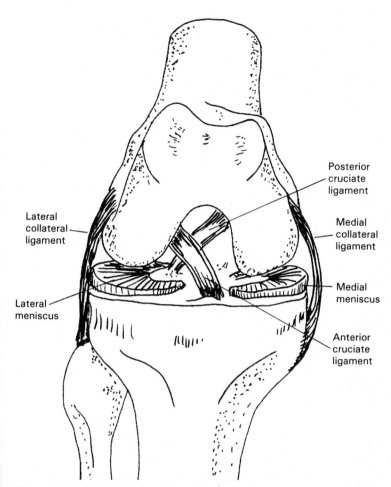

Figure 7.25 The knee joint. From the front, femur bent, showing cruciate ligaments, collateral ligaments and the menisci (cartilages).

The stability of the knee depends primarily on muscular support and on the action of the cruciate ligaments, and collateral ligaments, and to a lesser extent, the menisci (cartilages) (fig. 7.25).

The collateral ligaments (medial and lateral) are responsible for transverse stability during knee extension and the cruciates and collaterals together are responsible for antero-postero (forward and backward) stability, allowing the joint to work as a hinge.

During walking, running and working situations, the knee may be subjected to abnormal stresses. If stresses are too severe, a particular structure or structures will be damaged.

Diagnosis

Anyone who is responsible at any level for the care of athletes should know how to carry out a meaningful examination of a knee injury. It is sometimes possible to diagnose the exact damage to a knee if it is examined within half an hour after injury. This is before the reactions of inflammation, pain and swelling limit movement for diagnostic purposes.

History

In many traumatic conditions of the knee, the diagnosis may depend on the history alone. Thus the importance of taking a thorough history cannot be overstressed. The development of the symptoms is traced step by step from their beginnings to the time of consultation. The patient's assessment of how the condition or injury occurred, and even an onlooker's interpretation of the event, can be very useful.

Ask leading questions such as what was the patient's position at the time of injury; the direction of any extrinsic or intrinsic forces which may have been involved; and the presence or absence of locking, clicking and giving way.

Signs and Symptoms

1 Pain

The patient must be carefully questioned and tested to develop a clear picture to qualify and quantify the extent of the patient's pain. Pain at rest, pain on movement, on palpation and the way pain changes with time must all be recorded, and the strength and quality of the pain must be noted (for example, mild, throbbing, periodic and so on).

2 Swelling (water on the knee)

Swelling is a clear sign that the knee has been injured, although it does not always follow that the knee will become swollen after injury, particularly after minor meniscus damage.

If there is sudden swelling within half an hour after injury, this can generally be from haemarthrosis (bleeding into the joint). Slow swelling, up to 24 hours later, can be attributed to normal inflammatory processes.

If swelling persists after one or two weeks, the patient may self-diagnose a condition called "water on the knee". This is just a symptom of an underlying condition, and the best treatment is to discover and rectify that condition. However, draining off the liquid (a doctor's job, of course) is sometimes successful, as it may allow the underlying condition to heal more quickly. Removal of the fluid also allows a better contraction of the quadriceps, which then aids more fluid dispersion by forcing the fluid back into the system. This more efficient contraction also helps with knee strength and stability.

3 Muscular Atrophy

It is well documented that the strength of the knee joint is dependent primarily on the muscles which control it. While other muscles are involved, three major muscle groups act on the knee. The most important of these, both for strength and stability, are the quadriceps on the front of the thigh, and the hamstrings at the back, which add to knee stability. The third group is the gastrocnemius comprising the bulk of the calf muscle below the knee at the back. Thus, if there is any loss of muscular strength, power or endurance of these groups following a knee injury, the important consequence will be a corresponding loss of knee stability.

It is well recognised that muscular atrophy, or wastage, is a consistent symptom of knee injury, mainly because of disuse from pain and spasm. This is a matter of common clinical observation. This deficiency can easily lead to further loss of joint stability and further damage.

4 Locking

When testing for the presence or absence of locking in a knee joint, caution must be taken in accepting the patient's interpretation of "locking". He or she may regard stiffness or lack of movement caused from pain, fluid or scarring as meaning locking. True locking occurs where there is a sudden block in movement sustained by the mechanism of rotation while flexing or extending the joint. It may unlock just as suddenly, not gradually as from fluid pressure.

Locking can be a sign of meniscus damage as the injured or torn part of the meniscus becomes wedged between the femoral and tibial condyles (top of the tibia and bottom of the femur). However, locking may be exhibited also in some other conditions, such as a torn cruciate ligament, chondromalacia patella, epiphyseal separation, patella dislocation and osteochondritis dissecans.

Be aware also that absence of locking does not automatically indicate that there is not meniscus damage.

5   Precipitance

Precipitance is the sudden giving way of the knee during function. In effect, the quadriceps cannot support the knee joint as a result of some internal derangement in the knee itself. This may well be meniscus damage, ligament damage or irregular arthritic surface damage.

6   "Unstable Knee"

The term "unstable knee" is, of itself, not a diagnosis. The condition is a symptom which results from injury of one or more particular structures supporting the joint. The stability of the knee depends primarily on muscular support and on the action of the cruciate ligaments and collateral ligaments, and to a lesser extent the menisci (cartilages). Therefore, damage to any one or all of these structures may cause excessive movement in any direction, giving rise to an "unstable knee". The most common problem occurs when the medial ligament (and the anterior cruciate ligament) are damaged. When the player rotates on his or her knee, such as in changing direction, the femur shifts forward on the tibia and the knee gives way.

7   Loss of Function

Virtually any of the symptoms previously mentioned, no matter what the cause, may lead to a loss of function in the knee joint.

"Loss of function" is always linked with one or more of these preceding symptoms, although, to the patient, the importance of any other symptoms may be insignificant when compared to the functional disability which follows an injury. In fact, this loss of function may be the only reason for seeking treatment. That is, the patient may not be able to perform a particular action or movement, or participate in a particular sport or carry out a normal occupation. The patient cannot bend the knee because of pain or swelling or cannot walk without limping because of one

or more factors, or cannot run because a knee keeps "giving way".
Thus the symptom may be an important clue to establish the
direction which diagnostic investigation should follow.

Radiographic Examination

It is essential to X-ray knee injuries to rule out the possibility of
bone damage, chips, fractures and diseases of the patella and knee
joint.

Diagnosis of Specific Injuries

Ligaments

Collateral ligaments   The collateral ligaments strengthen the
articular joint capsule surrounding the knee joint. They are the
medial ligament on the inside and the lateral ligament on the
outside (fig. 7.25). These ligaments become taut during extension
(straightening) and slackened during flexion (bending). As such,
they are responsible for transverse stability while the knee is in
extension. The most common injury to the knee is damage to the
medial ligament, generally caused by a blow to the outside of the
knee causing stress on the inside (fig. 7.26).

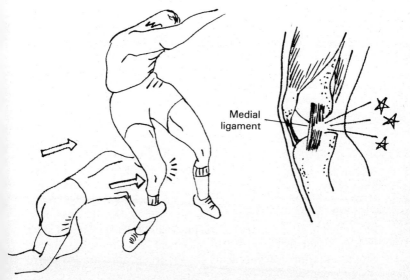

Medial
ligament

Figure 7.26   Action causing damage to the medial ligament.

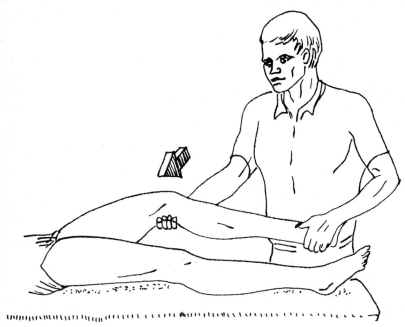

Figure 7.27   Testing for medial ligament damage.

The medial ligament sprain is tested with the knee in complete extension and at 30 degrees flexion. An inward pressure is applied on the outside of the knee while the ankle is supported. This will produce pain on the inside of the knee, generally at the attachment of the medial ligament to the femur or tibia (fig. 7.27)

The test for lateral ligament damage is the reverse of that of the medial ligament.

Cruciate ligaments   The cruciate ligaments lie in the centre of the joint, crossing each other (hence the name: cruciate means "cross-shaped". See fig. 7.25). There are two of them and they are mainly responsible for backwards and forwards stability; they allow the joint to work as a hinge.

The simplest way to damage one or both of these ligaments is to fall on the front part of the tibia (fig. 7.28). It is useful to know that a lesion (injury) of the posterior cruciate ligament leads to a posterior (backwards) displacement and similarly, a lesion of the anterior cruciate leads to abnormal anterior (forward) displacement.

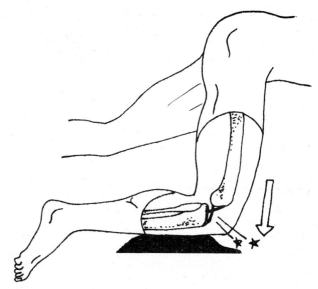

Figure 7.28 Injury to the cruciate ligaments. The femur slides on the tibia and damages the cruciates.

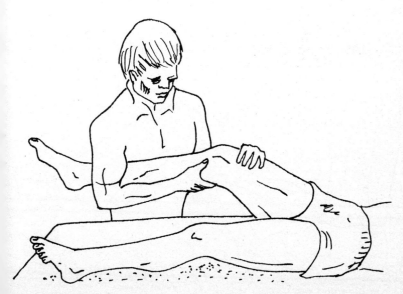

Figure 7.29 The Lachman test.

There are three tests for anterior cruciate ligament damage.

1 The Lachman test. Support the leg as in figure 7.29 and attempt to lift the tibia forwards on the femur. The test is positive if the tibia moves forward to a mushy soft end point. A stable knee will display no movement. (Compare with the other knee.)

2 Anterior drawer test. The patient lies on a table with the knee flexed to 90 degrees and the foot flat on the table, stabilised by the tester (fig. 7.30). Draw the tibia forward. An abnormal forward mobility by comparison with the other side indicates anterior cruciate ligament damage.

3 The crossover test. The patient stands upright with his or her feet together. The tester stabilises the injured leg. The patient then rotates his or her torso 90 degrees towards the injured side, crossing the uninjured leg over the fixed foot and planting it at a right angle to the fixed foot (fig. 7.31). As the patient contracts the quadriceps, he or she is asked to bend the knees toward the floor. The test is positive if the patient feels discomfort, precipitance, apprehension or can't do the test.

Posterior cruciate ligament   The posterior drawer test, carried out in a similar position to the anterior drawer test, can be a

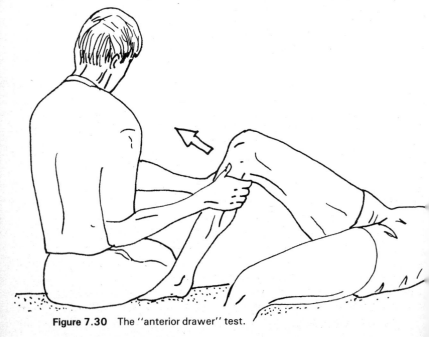

Figure 7.30   The "anterior drawer" test.

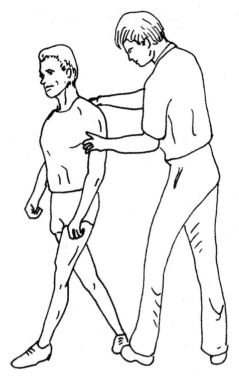

Figure 7.31   The ''crossover'' test.

reliable indication of posterior cruciate ligament damage. Ensure the tibia is centrally located on the femur (as compared with the other knee) and draw the tibia backwards. Excessive backward mobility indicates posterior cruciate ligament damage.

A second test is to compare the angle of the tibial tubercles when viewed from the side. If the posterior cruciate ligament is damaged, the tibia sags back spontaneously (fig. 7.32) to the posterior joint capsule. Raise the limb from the couch by the heel and note the degree of extension or hyperextension estimated (fig. 7.33).

Cartilage

The menisci, or cartilages, are half-moon-shaped pieces of gristle sitting between the tibia and the femur. There are two in each knee and their main function is to act as shock absorbers. They

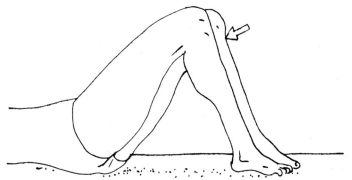

Figure 7.32 Torn posterior cruciate ligament — note the tibial head falls back when compared to the other leg.

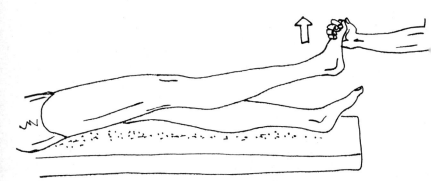

Figure 7.33 Test for posterior joint capsule strain.

also deepen the cavity of the socket for the femur to fit into. Their biggest drawback is their inability to regenerate if they are damaged, as they have a poor blood supply. For this reason, athletes fear the prospects of "doing a cartilage". However less than one per cent of knee injuries require an operation to remove a damaged cartilage.

Occasionally, if the cartilage is torn, and the torn shred resumes its original position (and function), no treatment may be necessary except routine pain relief and appropriate exercise. However, although the joint may be symptom-free for years, the torn cartilage may be displaced by a relatively simple rotary movement on the flexed knee. If the joint becomes continually painful and swollen, and if it locks or "gives way" regularly, strong

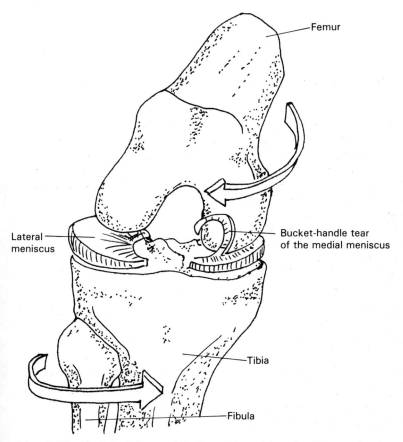

Figure 7.34   The knee is bent and the femur is rotating on the tibia, causing a tearing of the medial meniscus.

consideration should be given for the meniscus, or part thereof, to be removed (fig. 7.34)

Fluid and effusion are not always reliable guides to the diagnosis or severity of a meniscus injury. Neither is pain, as only damage of peripheral structures will register pain.

McMurrays test   There are many variations of this test and it can take experience for it to be meaningful. The knee should be bent to the greatest amount of flexion possible with the fingers and thumb placed over the joint line to detect "clicks" and "clunks" as the tibia is rotated to extremes on the femur (fig. 7.35). The

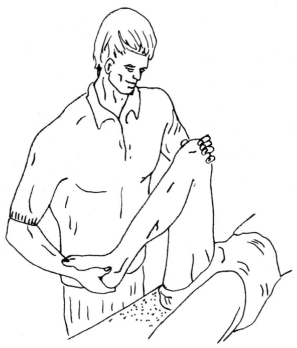

Figure 7.35   McMurrays test.

knee should flex past 90 degrees for the test to be useful. When positive, with good "clunks" resounding, the test is very helpful; when negative, it means little.

Bursae and Synovial Membranes

The bursa is a smooth, sac-like cavity which lessens friction and is lubricated with synovial fluid exuded by the synovial membrane. Overuse or direct violent contact can inflame and damage these structures. There is local tenderness, swelling and inflammation. Pain is usually present with tension of the skin in extreme flexion or under direct contact pressure.

Overall, it is difficult and often premature to offer an eager player a diagnosis and a forecast of the course of the injury after the first examination of an injured knee. When pain, inflammation and swelling have eased, by about the third day, a clearer picture may emerge.

Treatment of Knee Injuries

Virtually the same general treatment is given for all knee injuries. The main objectives are to:

- relieve pain and inflammation;
- control swelling;
- aid the healing of the sprain, tear, bruising or whatever the injury may be;
- regain and maintain musculature control of the joint by intensive exercise of the quadriceps, hamstring and calf;
- regain the full range of knee mobility;
- regain the full function of the knee, considering factors such as joint proprioception and walking, running, and other functional acitivities.

Early Treatment

The main aim immediately after injury is to keep bleeding and inflammation to a minimum, so ice, compression and elevation are applied as usual. After the joint has been taken out of ice (after about 20 minutes to half an hour), wrap a crepe bandage comfortably around the knee and advise the injured person to go home, keep his foot above the level of the heart, and begin isometric exercises for quadriceps and hamstrings. (Footballers rarely do this, their first stop is the pub or club until 10 p.m..) An extremely painful swollen knee is generally placed in a back slab (a kind of splint behind the knee to prevent movement), for two to three days until swelling has subsided and further assessment can determine the line of treatment.

Late Treatment

Regain strength The main therapy entails an intensive strengthening program for the quadriceps and hamstring muscle groups. The quadriceps, the large muscle group on the top of the thigh, strengthens, supports and gives control and stability to the knee joint, particularly when the ligaments (which normally help support the knee) are injured. Within three days of no exercise (because of pain), the thigh muscles of a fit footballer can waste by up to 3 cm in circumference. The three most important exercises are straight leg raising (fig. 7.2), knee extension (fig. 7.3 and fig. 7.36) and knee flexion (fig. 7.12).

Knee extension particularly works the vastus medialis, the "dew drop" muscle on the inside of the thigh just above the knee, which extends the knee the last 15 degrees. Be careful of pain from any patella injury while performing a knee extension. This exercise may have to be carried out with the foot rested on a chair below the table, straightening the leg only through the last 15 degrees of extension (fig. 7.36). In the beginning a rolled towel placed under the knee may be the best way to initiate this action.

Regain mobility   Knee mobility will increase automatically as the knee flexion exercise progresses. Different stresses can be applied, and further gains will be made with stretching, by doing squats, beginning with a partial squat and building up to a deep, full squat. However, squats should never be pushed past the limits of pain (fig. 7.4). It is unreasonable to expect people playing sports, particularly footballers, to be fully functional before they can manage a full squat. However, if full squats are carried out

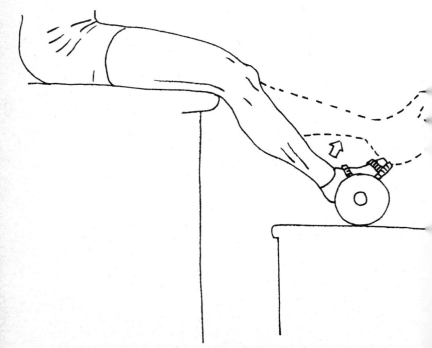

Figure 7.36   Knee extension — concentrating on the last 15 degrees.

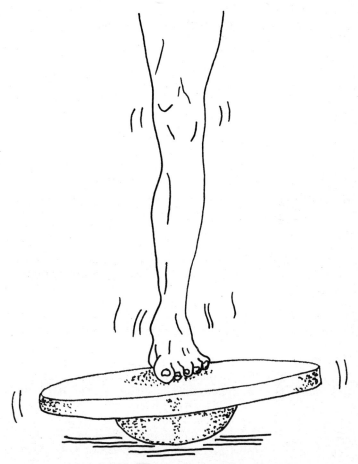

Figure 7.37   Improving proprioception by the use of a tilt board.

with heavy weights on the shoulder, an unnecessary burden is then placed on all joint structures, particularly menisci. It is never wise to perform squats with weights past halfway. Other knee mobility exercises are illustrated in figure 7.6 and in chapter 1, figure 1.3.

Regain proprioception   In a normal joint there is a nerve reflex system designed to act as a safeguard against damage from sudden severe demands. The muscles are kept in a state of "preparedness" to cope with these stresses. However, it has been found that when there is damage to the joint capsule, this nerve pathway is damaged also. So, because fewer nerve impulses are sent from the capsule to the muscles acting on the joint, the muscles are slow to respond and further knee damage may occur. Such aids as tilt boards and wobble-boards can improve these reflexes (fig. 7.37). Also, running in zigzag fashion plus training on the side of a hill in progressively smaller figures-of-eight will improve this proprioception fault.

Regain power An "isokinetic" retraining program should be undertaken to improve the power of the muscles controlling the joint. Sophisticated equipment is needed for these exercises. Power training can also be achieved with low to moderate weights using high speed contractions and large numbers of repetitions.

Regain function As soon as injured athletes can bear weight fully, they should start walking, leading up to jogging, running and then doing full sprints in a straight line. At about three-quarter pace, they may begin slow zigzags and then progress to quicker and sharper changes of direction, following by circles, stops, starts, figures-of-eight, ball dribbling and kicking, and finally all sport and team skills. They should not return to sport until they have demonstrated that they can perform all skills and training techniques at a full session of training, under playing conditions.

Prevention

The importance placed on the quadriceps and hamstrings in maintaining joint stability and influencing function has already been noted. Research and experience have shown that knee injuries are more likely to occur when these muscles become tired and not able to adequately control the joint. It is indeed very obvious then that an intensive pre-season and on-season strengthening program should be instituted and maintained to ensure sufficient strength, power and endurance for these main muscular supports of the knee joint.

There is some evidence that bracing may reduce the incidence and severity of ligament sprains, particularly for contact sports players whose game skills require twisting and turning.

At this stage, however, most braces with any metal or hard plastic constituents are illegal in Australian contact sports.

Strapping

It is impossible to strap a knee effectively to support a weakened structure and not lose a certain degree of flexibility, strength and co-ordination. Once the knee bends past thirty degrees the tibia rotates in its longitudinal axis and it is impossible to control this with strapping.

There are three circumstances where strapping may help a knee:

1 In the early stages of recovery from an injury, a crepe bandage will help to control swelling and give support.
2 For the actual game and training sessions, elastic adhesive tape provides psychological support. Simply wrap the bandage (tape) around the knee, leaving the kneecap free for full movement (fig. 7.38). A particular player may need this support for the first few games after injury.

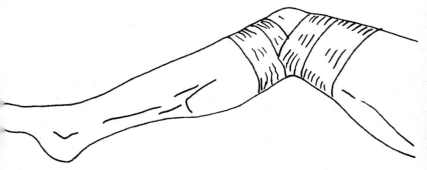

Figure 7.38   Figure-of-eight taping with an elastic bandage. This simple strapping is effective for most knee injuries.

3 To give support for certain ligament injuries. However, it is debatable whether the price of partial effectiveness is worth the loss of flexibility and control. These are generally complicated procedures and it is rarely worth the effort, although individual cases may benefit.

Generally, it is better to gain confidence in the leg by actually training on it instead of relying on props. It is unfortunately true also, in these days of tough professional sport, that by padding or strapping anything you are letting the opposition know you have an injury. For the amount of functional good that strapping may do, the player is probably better off strapping the other knee so that the opponents will kick that one instead.

ANKLE INJURIES

Soft tissue injuries to the ankle joint are very common among athletes and the lateral, or outside, ligament is damaged as much as five times as often as the medial, or inside ligament. In fact, with athletes, the lateral ligament complex of the ankle is the most frequently injured single structure in the body. This fact is important in understanding both the mechanism and prevention of the injury. Furthermore, because the ankle is a weight-bearing joint and closely associated with balance, if soft tissue injuries to this joint are treated incorrectly, or even lightly, the old adage "once a sprain, always a sprain" may prove correct.

Early and correct diagnosis is important and then a treatment plan specifically suited to the injury should be carried out. In this way, no soft tissue ankle injury should be a handicap to any athlete.

Anatomical Considerations

The ankle joint is between the talus, calcaneum, tibia and fibula and is normally stable because of its mechanical configurations and the support given by the ligaments (fig. 7.39). It is a modified hinge joint, with the talus acting like a ball-bearing within a mortice (fig. 7.40). A striking feature is that the medial and lateral ligaments are not symmetrical in size, shape or location. The medial ligament is a robust unit, whereas its lateral counterpart is made up of three distinct portions which vary in strength and thickness. This lateral ligament is clearly weaker mechanically then the medial ligament, and of the three portions, the anterior (front) one is the weakest. Furthermore, the higher arch on the inside of the foot tends to shunt stresses to the lateral side of the joint, which adds to the instability.

These factors, combined with the fact that there is very little muscular support on the front side of the ankle joint compared with the other side, predisposes the ankle to injury during body contact and "sidestepping" sports.

Cause

The ankle suffers a sprain when the ligaments are overstretched. This occurs most frequently when the foot is inverted, plantar flexed and internally rotated, placing the ankle in a most unstable position. A force from any direction with the foot in this situation may damage the ligament and joint capsule (fig. 7.41).

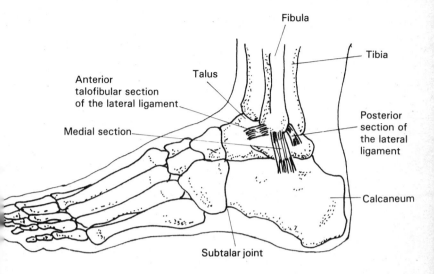

a. The lateral ligament complex of the ankle joint.

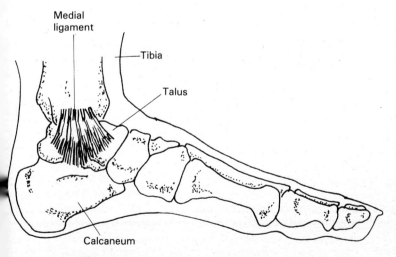

b. The medial ligament complex of the ankle joint.

Figure 7.39 The ligaments of the ankle.

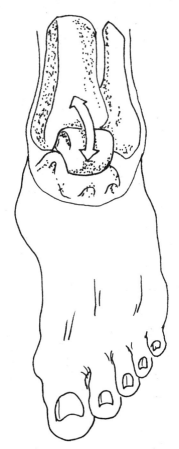

Figure 7.40   The ankle as a hinge joint.

Diagnosis

At the first possible opportunity, a significant ankle injury should be X-rayed to eliminate any damage to the bone. (A fracture is a rare occurrence, by the way.)

If squeezing the midshaft of the fibula produces pain at the ankle joint, this may well signify a fracture (fig. 7.42).

After appropriate questioning about the circumstances of the injury, and of the forces involved, it should be easy to compute the site of damage. Observation, plus palpation over the suspected area, will then localise the ligaments concerned. Finally, there are

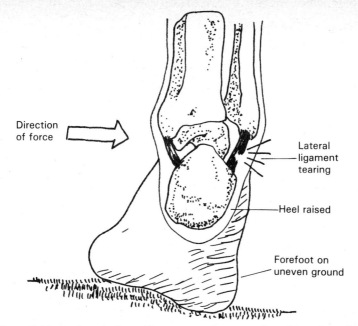

Direction of force

Lateral ligament tearing

Heel raised

Forefoot on uneven ground

Figure 7.41 Action of a lateral ligament sprain — rear view. Stress is applied while the heel is raised.

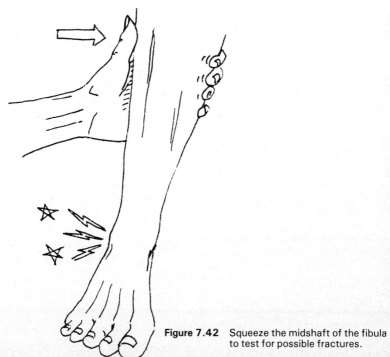

Figure 7.42 Squeeze the midshaft of the fibula to test for possible fractures.

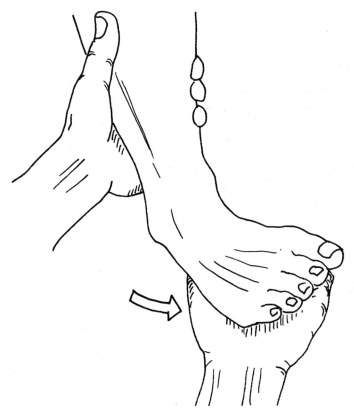

Figure 7.43 Inversion test. Stabilise the tibia while stressing the foot in inversion.

several stress and stability tests which should be undertaken by the health professional to gauge both severity of damage and any instability. The most common one to consider here is the inversion test (fig. 7.43).

The best time to carry out an examination is as soon as the patient is brought off the field of play and before severe pain, spasm and swelling limit effective diagnostic stress tests.

Treatment

Early Treatment

If a fracture is suspected, the player should be helped off the field of play, the leg splinted, then transported for X-rays and further treatment. Otherwise, the foot should be placed in a bucket of ice water or a cold pack of crushed ice applied in an effort to ease the pain and control excessive swelling. However, even if a fracture is suspected, this treatment will have positive effects and is still suitable. Because the ankle is pendant and therefore greatly influenced by the force of gravity, a comfortable crepe bandage should be wrapped around it to control the swelling, and the limb should be elevated (on a chair or pillow) to assist fluid drainage.

The ice treatment should be continued for at least three-quarters of an hour and can be repeated every three or four waking hours for the next 48 hours. Depending on the extent of damage and pain, weight should be kept off the joint and little or no exercise should be prescribed during this period.

Late Treatment

After the acute inflammation and pain have subsided, heat treatment can be started. This will continue to ease the pain, aid the healing processes (minimally) and increase tissue extensibility. This will increase the effectiveness of the exercise program which will follow the heat application.

Regain flexibility   Because of the natural tightness which occurs as a result of the scar tissue which replaces the injured ligament, the important first principle now is to regain the normal range of movement of the ankle and sub-talar joint (the joint below the ankle) (fig. 7.39(a)).

Exercises are begun with the foot off the ground (non-weight-bearing) and always only within limits of pain. The foot is gently moved through all ranges of movement, up, down, side to side and in circles.

Regain strength   As soon as pain permits, weight should be taken through the joint. Initially, share the weight through the good foot and or the hands, which are helping to support the patient on a convenient table or rails (fig. 7.44).

As the injury heals further, the patient should start on strong resistance exercises for the major muscle groups controlling the joint. First, standing with the toes on a doorstep and the ankles over the edge, the patient gives a complete stretch to the ankle joint and the calf muscles, followed by a complete contraction (tightening) so as to gain strength of the muscles (fig. 7.21).

Then second, with the feet placed about 30 cm apart, the ankle joint is gently rolled from side to side to gain lateral and medial

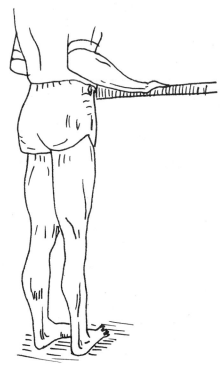

Figure 7.44   Gradually take weight on the damaged ankle.

mobility. The foot is moved into a position of stretch and held for 6 to 10 seconds. As the flexibility and strength improve more weight and stretch can be applied to the foot; always within the limits of pain (fig. 7.45).

Third, resistance should be applied to the dorsiflexors, the muscle group which pulls the foot back upwards. This will help to gain balanced foot and ankle musculature. A good technique is to resist the backward pull of the injured foot by pushing down against the foot with the other foot. An alternative method is to use a piece of rubber tubing (inner tube from a bicycle tyre perhaps) (fig. 7.46 a and b).

Regain power   An isokinetic retraining program should be undertaken as soon as the ankle joint is capable of accepting a resistance. The program should improve power of all muscles controlling the joint.

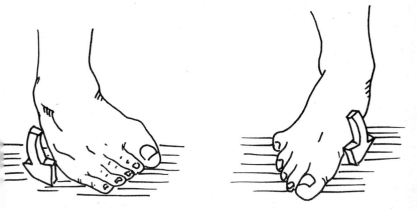

Figure 7.45   With feet placed 30 cm apart, roll ankles in and out.

Regain proprioception   In a normal joint there is a nerve reflex system designed to act as a safeguard against damage from sudden severe demands. The muscles are kept in a state of "preparedness" to cope with these stresses. However, it has been found that when there is damage to the joint capsule, this nerve pathway is damaged also. So because fewer impulses are sent from the capsule to the muscles acting on the joint (by way of the spinal cord), the muscles are slow to respond and further ankle damage may occur. Aids such as a wobble board can improve these reflexes (fig. 7.37). Running in zigzag fashion, plus training on the side of a hill in progressively smaller figures-of-eight, will improve the proprioception deficit.

Full Rehabilitation

The natural course from injury to full rehabilitation will follow a plan like this: flexibility exercises, leading to strengthening and weight-bearing exercises (including isokinetic exercises), leading to walking, to jogging, progressing to running at full speed in a straight line, then zigzagging, running backwards in circles, stopping and starting then in figure-of-eights on a hillside. At about the three-quarter pace running stage, sport-specific exercises and routines should be introduced, including controlled team participation and specific skills (such as ball work, team manouvres, jumping and so on).

The injured athlete should be able to cope with in at least one full session of hard training before resuming his or her sport, particularly if it is a body contact sport.

a. Resisting the dorsiflexors.

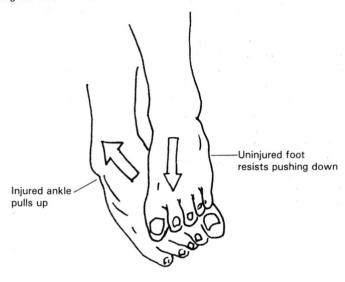

Injured ankle
pulls up

Uninjured foot
resists pushing down

b. Alternative resistance method.

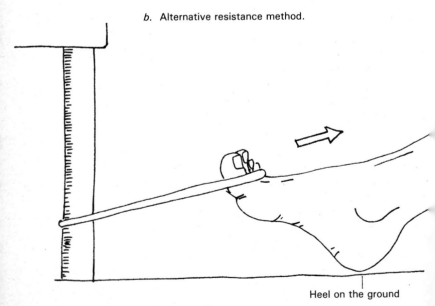

Heel on the ground

Figure 7.46 Dorsiflexor exercises.

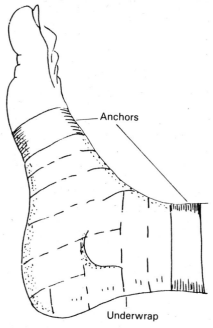

Anchors

Underwrap

a. Either shave hair to about 5 cm above the "ankle bones", or apply a foam underwrap and anchor it with zinc oxide tape.

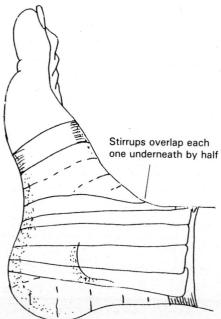

Stirrups overlap each one underneath by half

b. With the foot held at right angles to the tibia, apply 2 or 3 cm of non-elastic zinc oxide tape in consecutive stirrups under the arch.

Figure 7.47 Ankle taping.

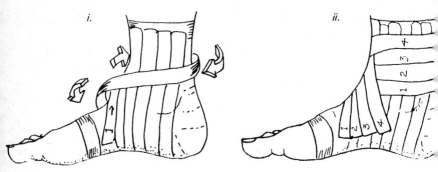

c. Use modified figure-of-eights to anchor the stirrups. Do not apply these supports tightly or they may irritate the Achilles tendon.

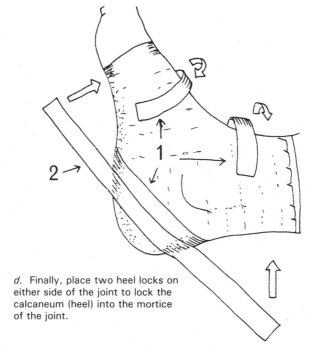

d. Finally, place two heel locks on either side of the joint to lock the calcaneum (heel) into the mortice of the joint.

Figure 7.47 Ankle taping (continued).

Prevention

Because of the anatomical and mechanical arrangement of the ankle joint, one would expect that it would be difficult to prevent this injury. However, it is possible to reduce both the incidence and severity of ligament damage simply with adequate conditioning in the first place, and second by taping the ankles in the appropriate way before competition.

Besides a general fitness program carried out in the off-season and pre-season and throughout the competition period, a specific training program should also be instituted for the ankle joints. This should stress gaining strength, endurance, flexibility, power and proprioception of the ankles in a functional manner, in much the same way as described above for rehabilitation. Special effort should be placed on heel cord stretching, as in the exercises in figure 7.21 and figure 7.22.

However, it is the authors' opinion that the most effective single measure to prevent ankle injuries is to tape both ankles correctly before every game and ideally before training as well. The aim of taping is not to prevent normal joint mobility, but to minimise excessive mobility without interfering with normal joint function. The tape simply acts as a second set of ligaments and in no way should weaken the joint or interfere with normal skills. Furthermore, if the ankles are taped this way, there is no additional stress placed on the knee joint (fig. 7.47).

Finally, there appears to be some evidence that ankle bracing can also help prevent the occurrence of ankle injuries. A properly fitted ankle brace placed over the sock has been shown to be effective in injury prevention. The obvious advantages with this method are the convenience of application, no necessity to shave the ankles and definitely more economy in the long run.

8
BACK AND NECK PAIN
IN SPORT

Pain originating in the spine is the most common affliction of the human race. Recent research reports that 80 per cent of the population of "civilised" countries will suffer from painful neck and back conditions at some stage of their lives. There is no specific category of subjects who suffer back pain more frequently than others; consequently athletes are not exempt from this malady.

To appreciate the management of back and neck injuries, including the cause, treatment and prevention, it is essential to understand some basic functional anatomy of the human spine.

ANATOMY

The vertebral column is composed of 33 bones (vertebrae) sitting on top of one another to form the spinal column (fig. 8.1). This column has a supportive, a protective and a locomotive function. The bony construction of the column allows for the attachment of many muscles and thereby is responsible for helping to maintain body form and shape. Protection is given to the vulnerable spinal cord which transverses its length and coupled with the attachment of the ribs between their constituent vertebra and the sternum, provides protection to the major internal organs of the body.

As the spine is composed of individual bones joined at specific points, great mobility of the human body is possible. The neck region is extremely mobile, allowing many complex combinations of movement. The lumbar region has fair mobility, with most movement occurring between the fifth lumbar vertebra and the immobile sacrum. The thorax, on the other hand, has limited movement because of the restrictions of the rib cage. Mobile regions of the spine are more susceptible to injury, therefore the cervical spine and the lower lumbar joints are the most frequently injured.

Each vertebra consists of a body from which a bony arch arises.

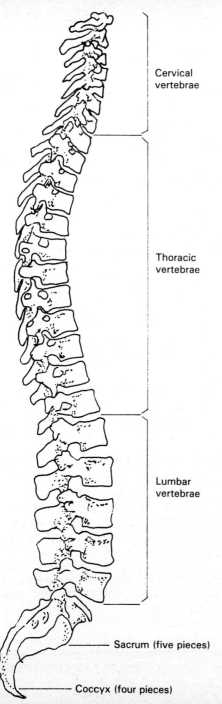

Cervical
vertebrae

Thoracic
vertebrae

Lumbar
vertebrae

—— Sacrum (five pieces)

—— Coccyx (four pieces)

Figure 8.1 The human spine.

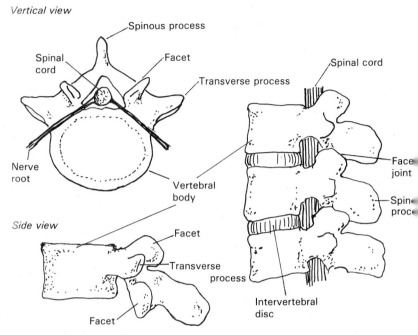

Figure 8.2 Diagrams of the spinal vertebrae and their bony articulations.

On each arch are articular processes which allow mobile joints called facet joints between each vertebra (fig. 8.2).

The facet joints are similar in construction to other major joints of the body. They are surrounded by a joint capsule and supported by ligaments. Therefore these joints are susceptible to soft tissue injury and degenerative joint disease (wear and tear arthritis) as are other bony joints of the body such as the knee, ankle and fingers.

A complex system of ligaments supports this flexible bony column (fig. 8.3). There is one anterior and one posterior longitudinal ligament lying along the length of the spine. In addition there are numerous smaller ligaments around the facet joints and between the vertebrae and their spinous processes. These ligaments provide the passive stability of the spine by helping to limit excessive movement and supporting structures such as the intervertebral discs. Active stability of the spine is maintained by the muscles of the back and neck (erector spinae) and the abdominal muscles.

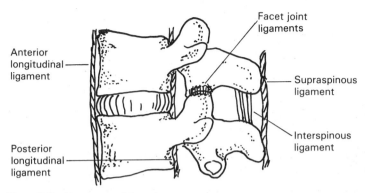

Figure 8.3 Ligaments of the spine.

Lying between the vertebral bodies are the intervertebral discs (fig. 8.4). Each disc is constructed of tough fibrocartilage rings (annulus fibrosis), which bind the vertebral bodies together and support the soft "gel" like nucleus of the disc. These discs facilitate movement of the spine, the nucleus acting as a ball bearing for rocking and rotational type movement. The nucleus also has the ability to imbibe fluid from its surroundings to control compression forces acting on the disc, therefore acting as a "shock absorber". With ageing, the ability to distribute fluids and counter compression decreases, leaving the disc vulnerable to degenerative changes and injury. The major cause of early degeneration appears to be related to our sedentary lifestyle. Bad posture, through prolonged sitting and little or no physical activity, will produce a progressive deterioration in the supporting structures and accelerate the ageing process. Continually lifting heavy weights and hard manual labour, particularly through a restricted range of motion, can also accentuate ageing changes to the spine.

Finally, the other important structures which may incur damage are the peripheral nerves. These peripheral nerves transmit messages, originating in the brain, from the spinal cord to the extremities (for example, movement) and from the extremities back to the spinal cord and hence the brain (for example, touch, pressure, pain, and so on). They leave the spinal column directly behind the posterior longitudinal ligament and facet joints. When damage occurs to these structures, or the disc is protruding, pressure is often placed on one or more of these nerves and the patient may experience symptoms of pins and needles, numbness, pain, unusual sensations, weakness and even paralysis in an extremity.

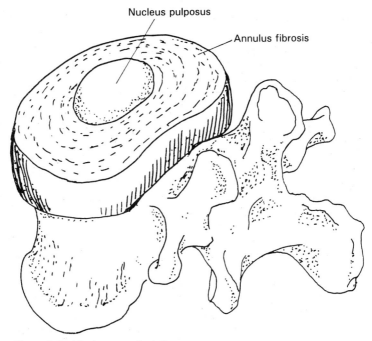

Figure 8.4 The intervertebral disc.

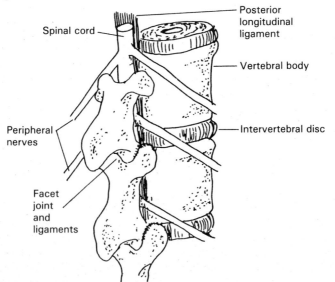

Figure 8.5 Side-rear view of the spinal column.

BACKACHE IN SPORT

No part of the human body has attracted more mythology or ignorance than dealing with the "crook back". There are many views available to the back pain sufferer. The medical scientific community still remains uncertain as to the precise cause of back pain and to the best management procedures. However, there are many practical guidelines and "proven" therapeutic techniques that can be followed to aid the unfortunate sufferer of back and neck pain.

Hypotheses as to the cause and treatment of back pain abound and while no unanimous opinion can be reached, there are two schools of thought in the community.

First, there is the "pseudoscientific" school, which supports the view that back pain and many other ailments are due to minor displacements of the bones of the spine and that adjustment of these displacements can cure the ailing back. At present there is no body of scientific evidence to prove this. While manipulative techniques can be effective in providing symptomatic relief and are used extensively by the authors, we are not convinced of their use in attempting to "readjust" spinal malalignment or "put displaced discs back in".

The second school of thought is that spinal pain is due to a wide variety of sometimes complex causes. Back pain can range from simple ligamentous sprains to the various diseases that affect the spine or its adjacent organs. Back pain sufferers often need the skill of many members of the health team, such as the family doctor, orthopaedic and neurosurgeons, the physiotherapist and the podiatrist to achieve a resolution of their problem. In this book we hope to present some fairly straightforward guidelines, based on scientific principles and our experience in the field, for the athlete who gets backache.

CAUSE OF SPINAL PAIN

Acute back pain in sport is usually due to the wrenching of soft tissues which support the spine. These soft tissue structures include the muscles, ligaments and the fibrous outer coating of the disc. Rarely is a bone broken or dislocated and if this situation does arise, catastrophic permanent paralysis often results due to spinal cord damage. Other bony injuries are more common. Landing heavily on straight legs may cause crushing of vertebrae. Vigorous repeated back movements (for example, rowing, gymnastics, fast bowling or weightlifting), may cause fatigue (overuse) stress fractures of the spinal arch of the vertebrae.

Most spinal injuries occur with sudden forward bending and twisting (flexion and rotation). These movements, when forced at speed, or by straining against a heavy lift, can place a stretching stress to one or more of the supporting structures of the spine, usually the ligaments or the fibrous outer coating of the disc.

This may occur when the sportsperson is, for instance, bending to pick up a ball, lifting incorrectly, pushing in a scrum, suffering a whiplash injury in a tackle or repetitive forward and sideways movement such as throwing. Sleeping is obviously non-violent; however, through lying heavily for hours on end on an improper pillow, or sleeping if overtired, drugged or inebriated, the poor position of the spine may induce injury. In healthy sleep a person will turn 40-60 times a night so that the 5 kg weight of the head is redistributed evenly.

In summary, most cases of back pain in sport arise from some mechanical disruption of the soft tissues that support the spine (for example, muscles, ligaments, disc, nerves). The resultant damage will lead to pain, inflammation and, as with all soft tissue injury, repair by *scar tissue formation* with its inherent inflexibility and weakness.

FACTORS WHICH MAY PREDISPOSE TO BACK PAIN

POSTURE

Poor posture is a major cause of overstress on the spine's supportive mechanisms. Good posture means the muscular and skeletal systems are in a balanced state which protects the structures of the spine against undue stress. Poor posture is a faulty relationship of the various parts of the body which produce increasing strain on the spine (fig. 8.6).

The normal spinal curves shown in figure 8.6(b) are designed to maintain the body form against gravity and to compensate for continual postural changes. The strongest mechanical postures are achieved by maintaining the lumbar and cervical lordotic curves in all positions of work or play. Once these curves are reversed, stress is placed upon the spinal joints.

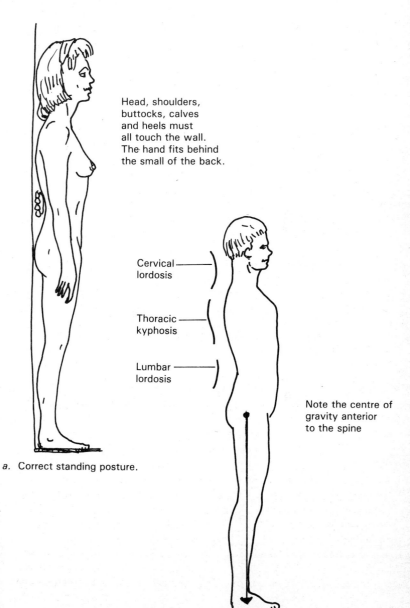

Head, shoulders,
buttocks, calves
and heels must
all touch the wall.
The hand fits behind
the small of the back.

Cervical lordosis

Thoracic kyphosis

Lumbar lordosis

Note the centre of
gravity anterior
to the spine

a. Correct standing posture.

b. Normal spinal curves.

Figure 8.6 Posture.

Sitting Posture

The commonest postural fault is incorrect sitting where the body slouches into a seat which does not support the natural curves of the spine. Poor sitting posture allows the spine to sag into reverse curves, particularly in the regions of the neck and low back (fig. 8.7). The line of gravity which, in the normal standing posture, falls anterior to the spine, now takes a line through the lower spinal joints. This situation produces a prolonged stretch to the ligaments of the spine and also dramatically increases the pressure inside the disc. It is this prolonged stretch over many years in the slumped posture that does damage, like stretching an elastic band to its extreme until it frays and weakens. Sports activity or simple everyday movements such as tying shoe laces, sneezing, bending over, and so on can cause acute damage to these already weakened structures.

Correct sitting involves attempting to maintain the natural curves of the body (fig. 8.8). A firm lumbar support is essential and a simple cushion can be an effective substitute. Advanced chair designs have recently led to a range of chairs that set an angle of approximately 130 degrees between the trunk and the thigh with some of the body's weight distributed to the knees.

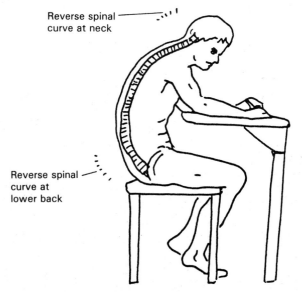

Reverse spinal curve at neck

Reverse spinal curve at lower back

Figure 8.7 Poor sitting posture.

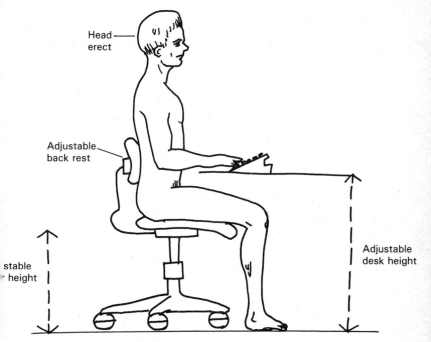

Head erect

Adjustable back rest

stable height

Adjustable desk height

a. Standard sitting posture.

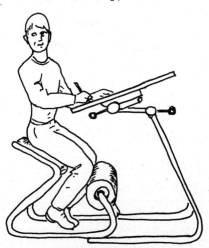

b. Advanced sitting posture
(Note the sloped desk (15 degrees)
to reduce the postural stress on
the neck.)

Figure 8.8 Correcting sitting posture.

This allows the maintenance of the lumbar lordosis and the line of gravity to fall in its natural position of anterior to the spine (fig. 8.8(b). In theory, this should be the most comfortable and least stressful position of seating.

Lifting Posture

Weightlifting has become an increasingly important part of almost all sports training. Therefore, correct technique and posture are essential to prevent injury. The back is capable of supporting considerable weight but is open to injury if the weight is excessive or if the angles of movement are mechanically insecure.

Lifting stresses are increased with the loss of the normal lumbar curve. The lumbar curve is lost by two postural faults, as shown in figure 8.9. First, a person may hold the weight away from the body, causing the lower back to bend. Second, the person may bend forward at the low back and pelvis to execute a lift. In these situations extra work must be done by the spinal muscles to complete the lift and protect the back. The pressure inside the disc also will increase to unacceptable limits in these positions. If the speed of the lift or the amount of weight lifted exceeds the strength of the spinal muscles, the muscles, ligaments or discs will be injured. The serious lifting injuries damage the disc structures

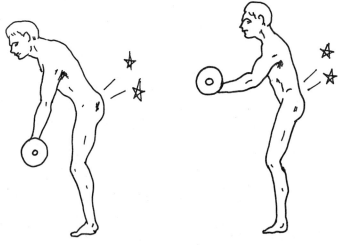

a. Back bent, instead of knees.   *b.* Weight held too far from body.

Figure 8.9 Poor lifting techniques.

and occasionally the bone. Most lifting injuries, however, are
ligament and muscle sprains and strains.

Correct lifting posture involves keeping the weight as close as
possible to the body. The back's "spring shape", especially the
lumbar lordosis, must be maintained by holding the back erect
with the knees bent. The lift is completed by using the stronger
thigh muscles to straighten the knees, not by lifting using the back
like a crane (fig. 8.10).

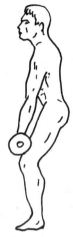

Figure 8.10   Correct lifting action.

(Note the weight close to the body; back straight, knees bent.)

The spine is supported during lifting by muscular action of the
spinal muscles and the pressure built up within the abdominal and
thoracic cavities. Muscles that attach to the spine move the spine
and support during the lift, but are not designed to actually carry
out the lift. The intra-abdominal pressure built up during a lift
serves to hold the spine erect under stress. The pressure is regulated
by the abdominal muscles in all lifting, bending and straining
movements of the spine. When heavy weight training is
contemplated, the use of a lumbosacral belt (kidney belt) can be
of assistance. The belt is not applied to support the joints and
bones, but to enhance the abdominal muscles in regulating the
abdominal cavity pressure to support the spine.

Common Postural Anomalies

Postural Faults

Observations of young athletes will disclose that very few individuals maintain correct postural alignment in either of the static positions of sitting and standing. Coaches tend to emphasise dynamic posture, especially in achieving the skill movements of sport. However, there is a tendency to overlook the importance of static postures maintained away from the sports field. Young athletes spend most of their time either sitting or standing, often incorrectly, leading to the development of postural faults. A postural fault is defined as a malalignment of the body which can be corrected by voluntary movement and corrective stretching.

The most common postural fault observed in athletes is the "sway back". This postural fault allows the pelvis to be rotated forward and down, hollowing the lower back. The shoulders are rounded with the head and neck protruding forward (fig. 8.11).

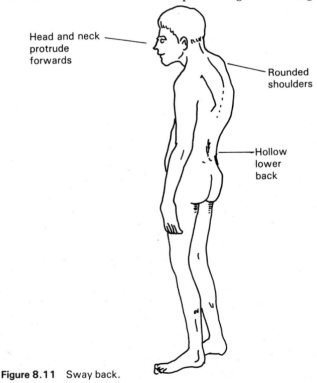

Head and neck
protrude
forwards

Rounded
shoulders

Hollow
lower
back

Figure 8.11   Sway back.

Poor posture, especially in sitting, and inappropriate exercises produce a shortening of the anterior muscles, tilting the pelvis and neck forward and putting uneven strain on spinal ligaments and discs. The back muscles tend to shorten to accommodate to this new position, causing a flexibility/strength muscular imbalance of the muscles controlling the pelvis and neck. Pregnancy or a large abdomen aggravates the problem by increasing the weight in front, especially if the abdominal muscles are weak. Table 8.1 depicts the specific tight and weak muscles for the clinician.

Table 8.1 Specific muscles involved in the strength-flexibility imbalance situations.

Tight muscle groups	Weak muscle groups
Lower body	
Triceps surae	Tibialis anterior
Hamstrings	Vastus medialis
Hip flexors: iliopsoas, rectus femoris	Gluteals
Tensor fascia lata	Hip abductors
Thigh adductors	
Piriformis	
Quadratus lumborum	
Low back extensors	
Tibialis posterior	
Upper body	
Levator scapulae	Serratus anterior
Upper trapezius	Rhomboids
Pectoralis major	Lower trapezius
Pectoralis minor	Deep neck flexors
Sterocliedomastoid	Extensors of the arm
Flexors of the upper extremity	

Lateral pelvic tilt and lateral curvatures of the spine (scoliosis) may occur due to postural faults and muscle imbalance (fig. 8.12).

The habitual resting stance adopted by the young with the weight on one leg will induce a lateral pelvic tilt. Mild scoliosis is common amongst young athletes who participate in unilateral sports such as tennis, throwing sports and rowing. Repeated movements of the spine during sport and training results in the back muscles on the dominant side of the body becoming more developed and stronger than on the other side. This strength imbalance causes a shift of the spine towards the stronger muscles. It is extremely important for coaches and parents of children in these sports to observe their posture and encourage regular

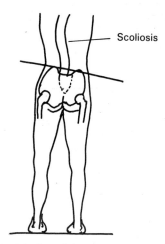

Figure 8.12   Lateral pelvic tilt and the compensatory spinal scoliosis.

exercise for the opposite side of their bodies to ensure equal development.

The long continued effects of minor postural faults coupled with the repetitive stress of training and competition will produce overstretching and weakening of the ligaments, making the spinal joints and discs more susceptible to strain. Forward and lateral displacements of the pelvis can reduce the efficiency of running and have a deleterious effect on performance.

Assessment and correction of postural faults and muscular imbalances should only be conducted by a sports physiotherapist or sports medicine doctor. A corrective program would involve treating the spinal pain, then putting increased emphasis on strengthening the weak muscles and stretching the tighter groups. The maintenance of proper posture and a balanced exercise program will help prevent the development of a postural fault.

Postural Defects

These are situations where the skeletal structure of the body has been changed due to disease, injury or hereditary factors and cannot be corrected by voluntary movement and stretching. Some correction may be possible with bracing, surgery or orthotic appliances.

Ideopathic scoliosis   This is a lateral curvature of the spine that can occur in approximately 5 per cent of all children. It is often first noticed by the physical education teacher, nurse or parent. The cause of this complaint in growing children is unknown. Scoliosis causes little discomfort or pain and does not preclude the child from sports or activity. All children with scoliosis must be examined by a doctor. Mild cases are kept under observation, while the more severe cases often need orthopaedic management with surgery, corsets and corrective exercises.

A compensatory scoliosis is always present when there is lateral pelvic tilt associated with leg length discrepancies. The short leg syndrome may be due to intrinsic causes such as congenital or hereditary defects in the growth of long bones, epiphyseal trauma during growth and pathological processes during growth. Extrinsic causes include traumas such as fractures and dislocations, leg alignment genu varum/valgum or secondary to unilateral foot pronation (see chapter 9, "Back, hip and pelvic pain in running athletes").

Round back   This postural defect is caused as a result of "Scheuermann's disease". This complaint affects adolescent boys; the vertebrae are improperly formed and become wedge shaped (fig. 8.13).

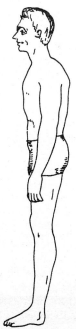

Figure 8.13   Round back caused by Scheuermann's disease.

The condition is usually symptomless and self-limiting in most cases. Individuals who have had the condition only become aware of it when it is picked up by chance X-ray of the chest or spine for other purposes.

In some cases the disease can cause chronic backache in boys, particularly when fatigued, for example, by sitting all day at school, or often undertaking heavy lifting activities. The common finding with round back syndrome is for the upper back to become very stiff and easily fatigued. The problem responds very well to manual therapy techniques and regular back rehabilitation exercises.

STRESS INJURIES TO THE SPINE

These injuries are usually the result of "overuse" (see "Overuse Injuries", part IV).

Overuse back injury is common in sports such as cricket fast bowling, javelin throwing, gymnastics, tennis and rugby. Damage is caused by shearing forces applied to a side bend and rotated spine such as when the leading foot strikes the ground during a fast bowling delivery (fig. 8.14).

Repeated activity coupled with a lack of fitness or poor technique will place accumulated stress on to the soft tissues that support the spine on the impact or leading side. This accumulated stress will eventually cause breakdown of these soft tissues, causing pain and inflammation. Continued activity will lead to a bony response to excessive stress; that is, a stress fracture (see chapter 9, p.267). When this type of fracture is of long standing, the defect is easily seen on X-ray and is termed a spondylolysis (fig. 8.15(a)). Early diagnosis is possible using a bone scan to pick up the stressed bone before a full fracture can occur.

A frank stress fracture may become a precursor to slippage of a vertebra forward in relation to the one below: termed a spondylolisthesis (fig. 8.15(b)). Spondylolisthesis may occur in sports which expose the back to heavy loads such as gymnastics, weightlifting, or diving, which can easily damage the growing adolescent. However, most spondylolistheses are primarily due to hereditary factors.

In most cases, sport can be continued provided the back is protected by the appropriate stabilisation exercises. Heavy weight-lifting and other activities which overstress the back in the forward bent position should be avoided. Growing adolescents with this

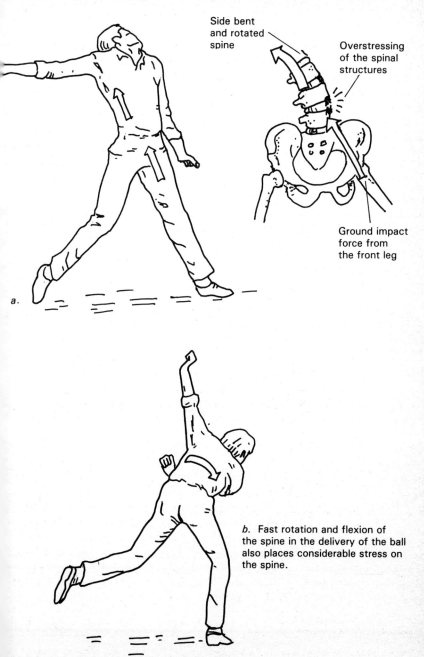

Side bent and rotated spine

Overstressing of the spinal structures

Ground impact force from the front leg

a.

b. Fast rotation and flexion of the spine in the delivery of the ball also places considerable stress on the spine.

Figure 8.14 Shearing forces applied to the spine during fast bowling.

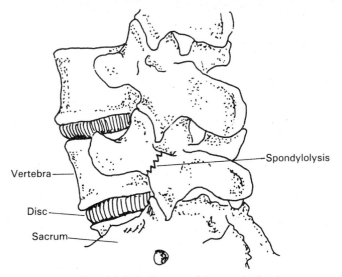

Vertebra

Spondylolysis

Disc

Sacrum

a. Spondylolysis: fracture of the vertebral arch.

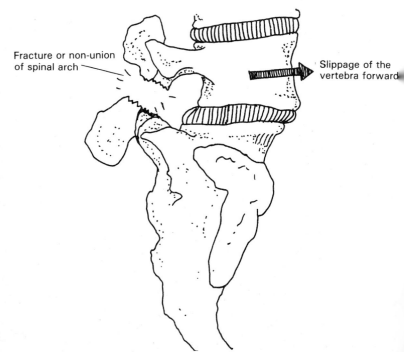

Fracture or non-union
of spinal arch

Slippage of the
vertebra forward

b. Spondylolisthesis: slippage of a vertebra.

Figure 8.15 Spondylolysis and spondylolisthesis.

condition should be closely monitored by their doctor. Persistent, unrelieved back pain or nerve compression may necessitate an operation to stabilise the slippage.

DEGENERATION *(wear and tear—osteoarthritis)*

Many older people who play sport may have osteoarthritis of the spine (fig. 8.16). This wear and tear process may have been caused by a number of factors:
- the ageing process;
- early injury which may have caused the joint to be unstable causing uneven wear and tear;
- an occupation which causes excessive stress in one area of the spine more than others, for example, clerical work sitting, heavy manual work in poor postural positions;

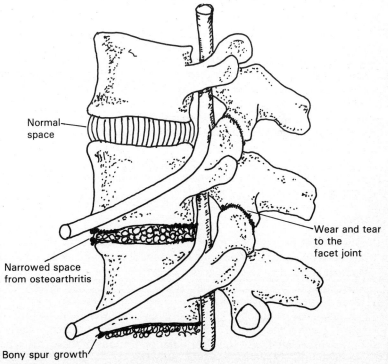

Normal space

Wear and tear to the facet joint

Narrowed space from osteoarthritis

Bony spur growth

Figure 8.16   The degenerative spine.

- the stresses of the sport itself, for example, early degenerative changes seen in the spines of rugby scrummaging forwards.

Osteoarthritis is often present when there is no discomfort at all. The chance finding of degenerative changes on X-ray should not deter activity. The degenerative spine, however, may be more susceptible to injury. Pain will generally arise from damage to the related soft tissues such as the ligaments surrounding and supporting the discs, and the spinal and peripheral nerves. This damage will eventually result in adhesions and scarring. At its worst, osteoarthritis narrows the discs and causes irritating bony spur growths on the vertebal bodies which can pressure the nerves producing pain and discomfort. Proper use of the spine, good posture and an appropriate balanced fitness program can significantly decrease wear and tear of the spine.

GENERAL HEALTH

Stress and Tension

Stress is a fact of modern life and can act as a trigger mechanism for spinal pain. Difficulties on the job, conflict in personal relationships, noise, grief, or exhaustion, coupled with the stresses of training and competing may force the athlete into a physical overload situation. As well as obtaining relief for the spinal pain symptoms, the athlete may need to re-evaluate his or her general lifestyle and training to look for ways to moderate stressors. Identifying goals and priorities, adequate rest and relaxation coupled with appropriate training and diet are important keys in controlling stress.

Diet

Overweight people have more chance of suffering back damage than fitter people. Carrying one kilogram of extra weight on your paunch is equal to five kilograms of extra weight applied to the ligaments and discs of the lower back. The desired target for body fat is 18 per cent in females and 12 per cent in males.

Conversely, improper diet, especially "fad weight reduction diets", can be disastrous for the athlete. The lack of energy and fatigue associated with the poor balance of foods in these "diets" can leave the athlete vulnerable to injury.

Fitness

There is ample documented evidence to show that both specific and general fitness helps prevent spinal pain. General fitness can lessen the risks by countering the onset of early fatigue which may leave the spine vulnerable to injury. Specific training of the spine should provide the athlete with the necessary flexibility, strength, power, endurance and agility for his or her sporting tasks.

MISCELLANEOUS CAUSES

Fracture

Violent trauma such as a direct blow to the spine or a spear tackle can cause breaks in the bony projections of the spine or in the vertebral bodies themselves. Serious injury often involves the spinal cord and nerves, resulting in catastrophic paralysis. The correct procedures for emergency management of these injuries are covered in part II, chapter 3.

Contusions

The spine is surrounded by thick muscle masses which are susceptible to direct blows causing damage, bleeding, swelling and pain within the muscle. These soft tissue injuries should be managed as are other muscle traumas such as the "corked thigh" (chapter 7, "Muscular injuries").

Pregnancy

To facilitate childbirth, a specific hormone is released which softens the ligaments of the lower back joints, sacroiliac joints and the symphysis pubis. This situation makes the female athlete more susceptible to spinal strain during and after pregnancy.

Following childbirth, it takes some months for these ligaments to regain their taut state and full strength. There are few contraindications to exercise during pregnancy; however, later in pregnancy, and just after delivery, the ligaments are in their weakest state, so heavy weight training and vigorous activity should be reduced. Full training should be resumed in slow, progressive steps coupled with an intense rehabilitation program to ensure the return to full strength and tightness of the back ligaments.

Disease

There are many diseases that affect the spine, such as various forms of cancer, ankylosing spondylitis and other inflammatory arthritic conditions. Diseases of other internal organs may have backache as one of their symptoms.

SIGNS AND SYMPTOMS OF SPINAL PAIN

As discussed previously in this chapter, most neck and back pain in sport has a mechanical origin. That is, there has been a mechanical breakdown of the soft tissue structures which support the spine due to one or more of a variety of underlying causes. Back pain has numerous labels which include: "lumbago", "fibrositis", "wry neck", "back out of place", and so on. The simplest descriptive term is back strain.

PAIN

A sudden forward or twisting motion may produce immediate pain in the areas damaged. With this quick onset the athlete will frequently give a history of being "unable to move" or of the back being "locked". The inability to move freely without sharp pain is caused by one of nature's immediate responses to injury called muscle spasm. Back muscles surrounding the damaged area contract into a tight spasm to act as a protective mechanism. This continued muscular contraction can be excruciatingly painful after a number of hours and definitely more so after a number of days. In some cases, the injured athlete may also experience referred pain in the hips, buttocks, groin or thigh, or the shoulder, shoulderblade, arm and chest with upper back and neck damage. If the peripheral nerves are involved, radiating pain and altered sensations may be present down the arm to the hand and fingers with neck injury and to the foot and leg with back injury. The thoracic spine may radiate pain and numbness around the chest wall and nerve irritation and muscle spasm can interfere with breathing.

Back pain may also have a slow onset. The athlete complains of a dull ache which is relieved by rest and aggravated with activity. When pain and symptoms are progressive it is usually indicative of a developing overuse syndrome. This slow onset will eventually lead to lasting pain and can also be associated to secondary muscle spasm, referred pain or the radiating pain and numbness of peripheral nerve irritation.

SWELLING

Secondary to all soft tissue injuries is swelling caused by the inflammatory process. Because of the confined space where the peripheral nerves leave the spinal column (fig. 8.5), any excess swelling from soft tissue injury may irritate these nerves. Symptoms may range from radiating pain down the leg/arm, pins and needles numbness to muscle weakness. These radiating symptoms are termed "lumbago" or "sciatica". As pain, swelling and muscle spasms subside, these symptoms should gradually lessen and disappear. If they persist it may be that the resultant scar tissue from the soft tissue damage is intertwined with the nerves; established degeneration and narrowing may irritate the nerves (fig. 8.16), or there may be an acute disc injury (see below). If sciatic, arm or chest symptoms do not subside with treatment within a few days, further investigation with X-rays, CAT scans and so on may be indicated.

DISC INJURY

Heavy loading of the spine such as lifting with a bent back, can cause damage and weakening of the outer coating of the disc (annulus fibrosus) which can then lead to the semi-soft inner core "bulging" or eventually rupturing out through the annulus to form a "disc prolapse" or disc "herniation" (fig. 8.17).

Disc injuries can occur at any age; however, they are more common in the older athletes. Discs slowly stiffen with age, lose their resilience and shrink, therefore becoming brittle and likely to rupture. Pressure inside the discs is least when lying, increases with standing, and is very high when in a slumped, sitting position or when the spine is bent forward under load.

Injury occurs when the pressure inside the disc is greater than the ability of the outer coating of the disc to absorb. Fissuring and tearing of this fibrous coating occurs, allowing the soft inside material to bulge outwards. In more advanced cases, the nucleus pulposus ruptures right through the wall. This situation used to be called a "slipped disc", but because of the false belief that slipped discs can be put back into place the term "disc prolapse" or "herniation" is preferred.

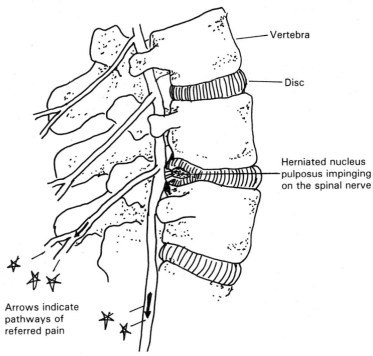

Vertebra

Disc

Herniated nucleus pulposus impinging on the spinal nerve

Arrows indicate pathways of referred pain

Figure 8.17 Disc bulge and eventual disc prolapse.

The prolapsed disc pulp can either press on the spinal cord, the peripheral nerve root or between the two nerve bundles without causing nerve damage (fig. 8.18).

Disc injury occurs more frequently in the lumbar spine, occasionally in the cervical spine and rarely in the thoracic spine. There are few pain endings in the discs themselves, therefore most pain is caused by pressure on adjacent tissues. Pressure placed on the peripheral nerves causes radiating pain, numbness and weakness in the areas supplied by the nerve. Fragments of the disc may be unstable and shift, causing changing or recurring symptoms. Symptoms include severe back pain and spasm, radiating pain, numbness, pins and needles, decreased tendon reflexes (for example, knee jerk), and weakness of muscles.

Most patients with so-called slipped discs do well with non-surgical treatment as described in this book. These injuries are essentially soft tissue damage and will heal in time. However, a small percentage may require surgery.

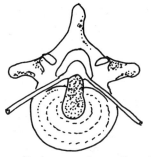

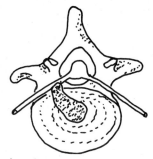

a. Nucleus pressing on the spinal cord.

b. An alternative situation — nucleus pressing on an emerging peripheral nerve root.

Figure 8.18 Disc prolapse.

LIMITATIONS OF FLEXIBILITY AND STRENGTH

Mechanical back injuries (including disc injury) are of soft tissue origin and, as discussed consistently throughout this book, heal by the process of laying down a scar. The drawback to this repair process is the tendency of the scar to contract and deform and become rigid and weak. Therefore, if the appropriate treatment is not followed, the damaged spine never fully regains its normal flexibility and range of motion. Further, it has been shown that unless properly exercised when forming, the scar tissue never approaches the strength of tissues it replaces. Therefore, injured backs become chronically inflexible and chronically weak if not rehabilitated correctly.

In reality, most spinal pain sufferers are inadequately rehabilitated and suffer the inevitable consequence of recurring pain and disability due to poorly healed ligaments and discs. The key to the successful treatment and prevention of back pain is the return to adequate strength and flexibility of the spine and its supports.

TREATMENT

1 PAIN AND SPASM RELIEF

First Aid

The appropriate first aid modality, as with all soft tissue injury, is R.I.C.E. using the methods described in part II, chapter 3, "Immediate treatment of soft tissue injuries", of this book. Severe pain and muscle spasm often gain relief with the application of moist heat. At home, hot water bottles, a hot shower, ray lamps and gentle massage all help to relieve pain and spasm.

Medical

The doctor can prescribe various drugs in this stage to help alleviate symptoms. Analgesics such as aspirin through to stronger prescription painkillers are helpful. Muscle relaxants and anti-inflammatory drugs may also be prescribed in severe cases.

Reduced Activity

Most back strains settle within 24 to 48 hours with rest. As soon as the patient can achieve reasonable movement without severe pain and spasm active treatment should be sought. Complete bed rest is often required for the severe injury and disc rupture. This means lying flat, or in the low back rest position (fig. 8.19).

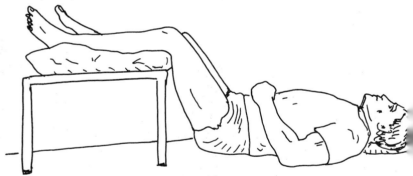

Figure 8.19   The low back rest position.

Sitting or lying propped up on pillows causes an increase in the pressure on the lumbar discs and ligaments causing aggravation of the symptoms. Within 5 to 10 days the patient has usually recovered sufficiently to allow a more active treatment regime. With cervical spine injuries a soft collar may be helpful in supporting the neck until symptoms subside.

Physiotherapy

The physiotherapist can offer a variety of physical treatments to help reduce pain and spasm. Many electrotherapeutic modalities are available; the selection and dosage require training and skill.

Manual therapy techniques of manipulation and mobilisation practised by trained therapists are useful at this stage. Contrary to popular belief, manipulative techniques do not "put back" supposedly misplaced bones, discs, joints, or realign the spine. The main effect of these techniques is to reduce muscle spasm and pain via complex reflex arcs and restoring movement to stiff painful joints.

Traction can be applied to stretch the vertebral column and its supports in the longitudinal plane to help relieve spasm. Traction may also help reduce interdiscal pressure, thereby relieving the radiating symptoms due to pressure on the peripheral nerves. Recent interest in inversion devices has prompted many athletes, gymnasiums and private individuals, with or without back pain, to purchase this type of equipment to gain the proposed benefits of hanging upside down (fig. 8.20).

Manufacturers of this equipment have made many grandiose claims about the positive effects of inversion. Such claims include the statements that it increases flexibility, retards ageing, reduces blood pressure, improves circulation, offers relaxation and relieves

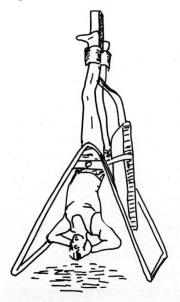

Figure 8.20 Inversion traction.

back pain. Some manufacturers also advocate that the apparatus can be used to promote physical fitness and as a muscle strengthening device. There is little or no scientific evidence to support any of these claims. However, with practical use of the device some benefits can be seen clinically.

It is probable that inversion will aid flexibility by applying a stretching force to the ligaments and other soft tissues supporting the spine. However, as this "stretching" is only in one plane, hanging upside down will only enhance, not replace a well balanced flexibility exercise program.

Physiotherapists and doctors have, for many years, recognised the beneficial effects of traction in the relief of pain from spinal origins. Many scientific studies have been undertaken to explain why this relief occurs, but no one reason is dominant. Inversion therapy is one method of providing traction to the spine and in our experience it can relieve back pain, particularly the discomfort experienced after training or competition. Hanging upside down is not a panacea for the treatment of back ailments. Most back complaints suffered by athletes are soft tissue problems, affecting the ligaments, muscles and tendons that support the spine. Therefore, managing these problems with inversion therapy alone is not enough. It should be used only in conjunction with other therapeutic modalities, especially a well designed strength and flexibility exercise program.

The most disturbing claim of manufacturers of inversion appliances is that this therapy has an effect of reducing blood pressure. Recent research in the United States has in fact shown that the opposite occurs. This study has demonstrated that there is a significant increase in blood pressure while the body is inverted. Therefore, many people are being inverted with little knowledge of the possible consequences. Inversion may be very dangerous for hypertensive or borderline hypertensive persons (people with higher blood pressure than normal).

Some manufacturers are recommending fitness and strengthening exercises in the inverted position. Exercise will increase blood pressure and exercise in the head-down position will increase blood pressure to unacceptable limits even in fit, healthy athletes. This increased pressure has been known to detach retinas from the back of eyeballs.

Summary for Inversion Traction

Uses

- It can assist in the relief of musculoskeletal pain after athletic activity.
- It is an adjunct to other therapies in the relief of pathological back pain.

Cautions

- Care must be taken to monitor the blood pressure of all people being inverted.
- Any untrained individual or an individual with suspected high blood pressure (overweight, smoker, over thirty and so on) must have a medical examination to establish circulatory status before inversion.

Contraindications

- Any hypertensive individual (increased blood pressure).
- All exercises in the head-down position.

Unfortunately, most patients and many practitioners equate symptomatic relief with healing. Pain, inflammation, swelling and spasm (the symptoms), usually abate within about ten days. However, the healing process is by no means complete. Soft tissue healing is not achieved until about four to six weeks or up to three months in the more severe injuries such as disc lesions. Once pain relief has been achieved, it is extremely dangerous to return to normal activity until a complete rehabilitative program has been completed. This is because the healing tissues have not regained their flexibility and strength, and the muscles and other soft tissues have lost their tone due to pain and inactivity and consequently are not as strong as before injury.

2   REHABILITATION

The rehabilitative program is divided into four stages and should be supervised by a sports physiotherapist.

The stages are:
(a) Correction of the underlying fault.
(b) Regaining complete flexibility of all muscles and joints associated with spinal movement.

(c) Regaining strength, power and endurance in the spine, trunk and abdominal muscles.
(d) A graduated return to function and sports.

Each stage must be completed to achieve a pain-free return to training and sports competition.

(a) Correction of the Underlying Faults

Many sports injuries are caused by incorrect technique/style. For example, fast bowlers or javelin throwers who have a "front on" delivery are more susceptible to low back injury than those with the "side on" style. Correct coaching in the proper skills and techniques of sport is essential to prevent injuries. If injury occurs, coaches and sports physiotherapists should work together to analyse and correct the incorrect technique of the athlete.

Back and neck injuries are often caused or aggravated by improper exercises conducted in training or in fitness programs. Aerobic classes and gyms can be a potential risk area when unqualified instructors prescribe inappropriate exercises for their clients. Exercises which place the spine at risk are illustrated in table 8.2. Injury occurs when incorrect exercises are performed at high speed with repetitive bouncing at the end of the range to the beat of rock music.

Athletes tend to do thousands of sit-up-type exercises to gain abdominal strength to help prevent back injury. However, most of these exercises involve bending forward at the hips which develops strong hip flexor muscles which tend to tilt the pelvis forward. As a result there is an increased curve forward in the lower back. This situation will lead to stretching and weakening of these structures and make them more prone to injury. Proper abdominal strengthening techniques are discussed below (fig. 8.23).

Minor postural deviations, muscle imbalances and other parameters discussed previously can lead to spinal injury. The assessment and correction of these spinal faults and muscle imbalances must be carried out by a competent sports physiotherapist. The workplace, sitting posture, bed, pillows, and any other relevant factors must be included in this assessment. Precise exercise prescription is needed to maintain these corrections.

(b) Regaining Complete Flexibility

The flexibility of the healing scar and the associated soft tissue structures of the spine is achieved by two means, namely:

Table 8.2 Examples of exercises which place the spine at risk.

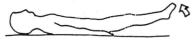

a. Double leg raise.

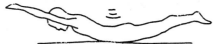

b. Hyperextension of the spine.

These exercises develop excessive pressure in the lower lumbar discs.

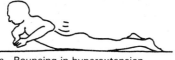

c. Bouncing in hyperextension.

These exercises can be performed safely at a slow, controlled speed. Fast, jerky movements, especially bouncing movements to music, can easily sprain the lower back or neck.

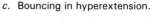

d. Cat variation.

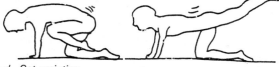

e. Toe touch.   *f.* Plough.

Flexing the spine into forced positions unlocks the spinal curves and places the spinal ligaments at risk — especially with bouncing, jerky movements.

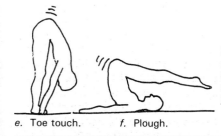

g. Sit-ups (incorrect).

The ordinary sit-up strengthens the hip flexors, which places strain on the lumbar ligaments by increasing the forward tilt of the pelvis.

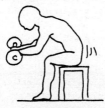

h. Bending weights.

Any bending of the trunk forward with weight can place an excessive load on the spine.

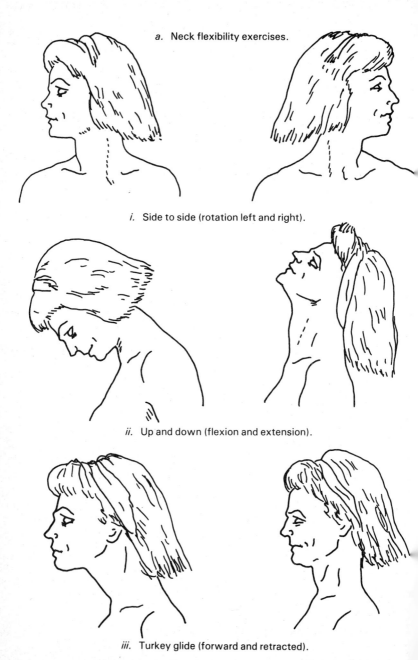

a. Neck flexibility exercises.

i. Side to side (rotation left and right).

ii. Up and down (flexion and extension).

iii. Turkey glide (forward and retracted).

Figure 8.21 Spinal flexibility exercises.

b. Thorax flexibility exercises.

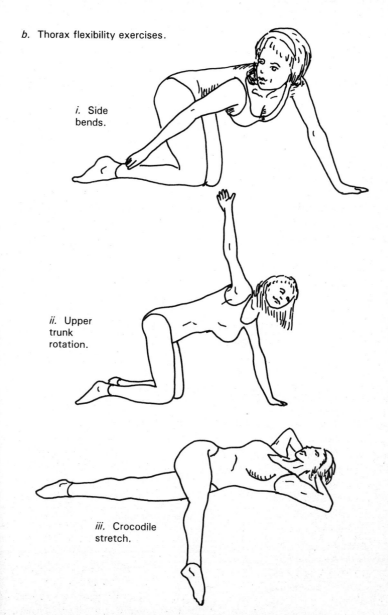

i. Side bends.

ii. Upper trunk rotation.

iii. Crocodile stretch.

Figure 8.21 Spinal flexibility exercises (continued).

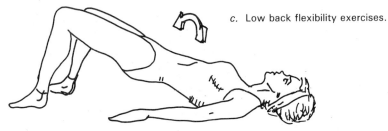

c. Low back flexibility exercises.

i. Bridge, then twist sideways each way.

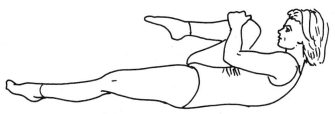

ii. Knee to chest, each knee.

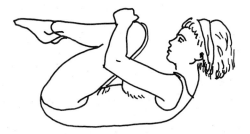

iii. Then double knees to chest.

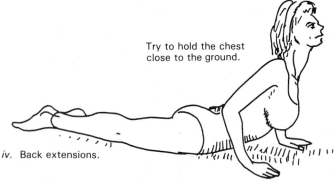

Try to hold the chest close to the ground.

iv. Back extensions.

Figure 8.21 Spinal flexibility exercises (continued).

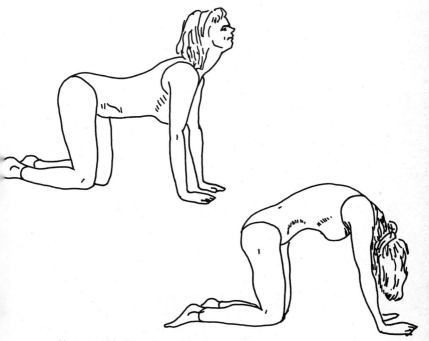

v. Humps and hollows (cat stretch); suitable for neck, thorax and low back flexibility.

Figure 8.21 Spinal flexibility exercises (continued).

physiotherapy skills and specific flexibility exercises. The physiotherapy skills include the various manual and manipulative techniques to increase all movements of the spine, particularly at individual spinal levels. Spinal flexibility exercises are then prescribed *within the limits of pain* to maintain and gain spinal ranges of motion. Examples of flexibility exercises are shown in figure 8.21.

Flexibility for muscles that act on or influence the spine must not be neglected in rehabilitation. Once muscle imbalance situations have been assessed and corrected, a general flexibility program must be devised for muscles such as the hip flexors, hamstrings, iliotibial band and the calf muscles. Some examples of stretches to these muscles are shown in figure 1.3.

(c) Regaining Strength

The basic concepts in regaining back strength are:
- abdominal muscle strength and control of the pelvis;
- regaining strength of the damaged soft tissues, trunk and hip extensors.

Pelvic control is gained by the pelvic tilt exercise, figure 8.22. The pelvis is voluntarily rotated forward, flattening the spine against the ground, holding this position for six seconds. This exercise forms the basis of many spinal exercises, especially the abdominal curl.

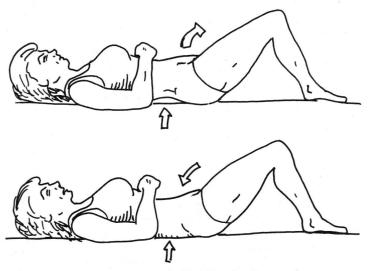

The pelvis is rotated, forcing the back flat onto the ground.

Figure 8.22   The pelvic tilt.

The abdominal curl is the best exercise set to increase strength of the abdominal muscles. If the exercise is performed correctly, the hip flexors will be inhibited, preventing strain on the back and isolating abdominal muscle action.

The athlete lies with knees bent and feet flat on the ground. A pelvic tilt is performed, the hamstring muscles are contracted and the feet held firmly to the ground, then the shoulders and upper back are curled off the ground to approximately 30 degrees (fig. 8.23(a)). If the lower back is arched forward, the trunk is higher than 30 degrees or the feet lift off the ground, the exercise

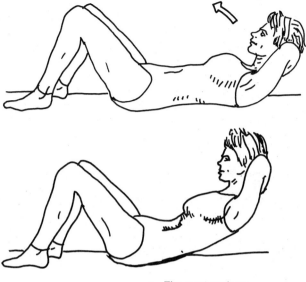

a. The correct sit-up.

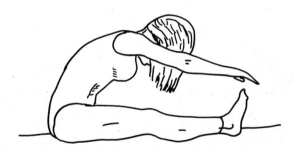

b. The incorrect sit-up.

Figure 8.23   Sit-ups.

is incorrect as these situations indicate that the hip flexors are being used (fig. 8.23(b)).

Abdominal curling can be extended as an exercise by a number of methods. Adding rotation of the trunk will strengthen the abdominal oblique muscles. Performing the exercise on an incline board and/or adding weights to the chest will increase the resistance.

To gain complete, strong healing of the damaged spine, the damaged soft tissues must be exposed to progressive strengthening

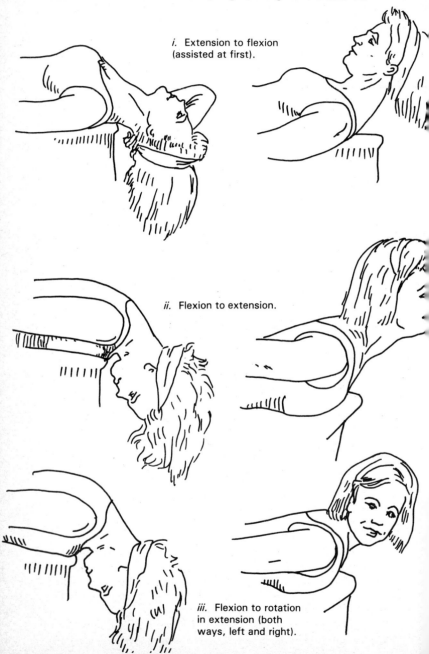

a. Resistance exercises for the neck, to gain strength and endurance.

i. Extension to flexion (assisted at first).

ii. Flexion to extension.

iii. Flexion to rotation in extension (both ways, left and right).

Figure 8.24 Spinal strengthening exercises.

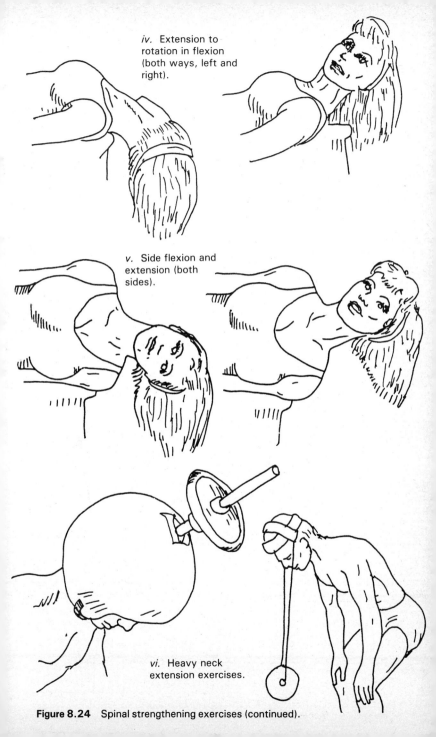

iv. Extension to rotation in flexion (both ways, left and right).

v. Side flexion and extension (both sides).

vi. Heavy neck extension exercises.

Figure 8.24 Spinal strengthening exercises (continued).

b. Resistances exercises for the low back and thorax.

i. Flexion to extension.

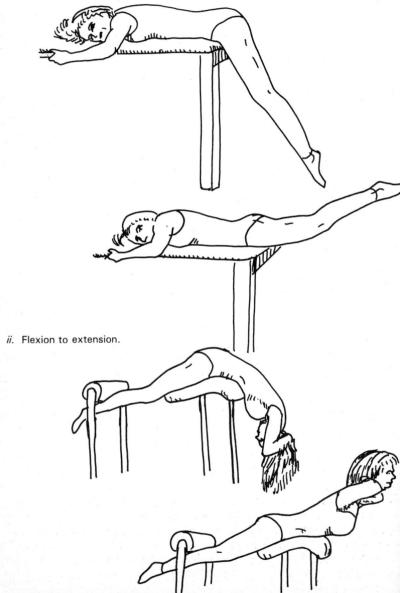

ii. Flexion to extension.

Figure 8.24 Spinal strengthening exercises (continued).

iii. Rotation in flexion to extension.

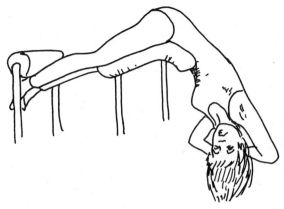

N.B. To increase strength, add weight behind the head.
To increase endurance, increase the number of repetitions.

exercises to achieve a mature scar. These exercises must be performed *within the limits of pain.* Progression is made until 20 repetitions are achieved, then progressing to the harder resistance exercises. Rotation of the trunk and weights can be added if heavy resistance training is required. Figure 8.24 depicts a selection of spine strengthening exercises.

Exercises that strengthen the back in the actions of sports are often needed to complete the strengthening program. Examples include using a rowing machine, or pulleys and weights or surgical rubber to provide resistance (fig. 8.25).

(d) Graduated Return to Function and Sports

As soon as symptomatic relief has been achieved and rehabilitation commenced, injured athletes must begin to regain their normal fitness. They should commence retraining for their lives, jobs and their sport. The most common mistake is to equate pain relief with healing and attempt to begin training/competition only to have the symptoms return. No specific formulae can be given for healing rates. Recovery depends on many factors such as the severity of injury, the structures involved, the quality of treatment and so on, and may last from a few weeks to three or more months.

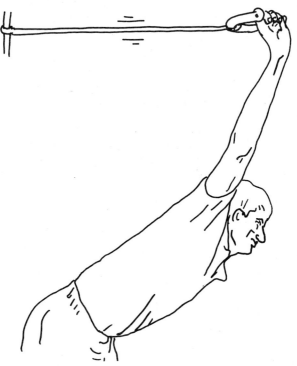

Figure 8.25 Surgical rubber used to provide resistance for the bowling action.

The best way to regain skills for a particular function is to start training lightly and then build up gradually; once again, always to the limits of pain. In the early stages of functional rehabilitation, swimming can be a valuable aid because the buoyancy of water allows for easier mobility of the trunk and limbs. It also aids functional retraining of the neck and back improving flexibility and strength, plus giving spinoff benefits to the cardiovascular system and general fitness. However, as we do not live in the water, swimming should only be an interim or complementary activity until exercise related to sport and work can be commenced.

It is imperative that the back rehabilitation program is maintained daily for at least six weeks after symptomatic relief to ensure a strong, mature scar. After this time, it is essential to continue with back exercises as part of the regular training program. If back exercises are allowed to lapse on regaining a symptom-free condition, back pain will inevitably return.

Prevention of back pain should incorporate the following principles:
- ensure good posture, both during exercise and in daily living;
- ensure good sporting technique and body mechanics;
- improve flexibility of the spine and the postural muscles which act on the spine: hamstrings, calves, hip flexors;
- maintain the strength of the trunk muscles and the muscles acting on the spine: the abdominals and hip extensors;
- maintain a balanced training program which includes a low back program.

PART IV
OVERUSE INJURIES

Human movement is achieved by muscles exerting force on rigid levers (bones) which are connected by joints. Therefore, motion is achieved by mechanical principles and just like any machine the human body is susceptible to breakdown. These breakdowns are termed overuse syndromes. They can occur in any part of the body that is exposed to intermittent stress over a period of time. An overuse injury may develop from one sustained period of activity, or from cumulative periods in the course of training or participation in sport.

Overuse syndromes usually manifest themselves in two ways:

- Cumulative stress on soft tissues will cause repetitive microtrauma, which causes irritation and eventual inflammation. This process will disturb tissue nutrition and cause eventual cell death, resulting in tissue repair by scar tissue formation.
- Bone responds to excessive stress by microfractures called "stress fractures" or by the overformation of bone, for example, "heel spur" (p.255). This overgrowth of bone is called an exostosis.

CAUSES OF OVERUSE SYNDROMES

The factors which lead to overuse injuries occurring can be grouped together into three broad categories:

- training errors;
- anatomical factors;
- environmental factors.

TRAINING ERRORS

Error in training technique is the single most common cause of injury. Doing "too much too soon" is a sure way of developing an overuse syndrome. Common faults in training programs are:

- Upgrading training levels too quickly. As a rule of thumb, the human mechanical system can stand an increase in load/activity of about ten per cent per week.
- Resuming training at too high a level after a layoff.
- Changing style, technique or equipment.

Stress is cumulative; therefore good training programs must allow for hard-easy days. Heavy sessions should occur only three or four times a week, with light workouts in between. This gives the body time to rest and recover from intense effort. Athletes must learn to listen to their bodies, as pain is nature's way of telling that injury and damage is occurring. The purpose of training is to expose the body to repeated stress, therefore the science of training is to know how much hard work the body can handle before it breaks down. If pain is experienced during a hard workout, the appropriate remedy is to reduce the intensity of the next few workouts so that no discomfort is felt on activity, then gradually increase the load until the required level is regained. Pain that persists after a workout, when the body is at rest, must receive the appropriate first aid (chapter 3) and should be checked by a qualified practitioner (sports medicine doctor or sports physiotherapist).

ANATOMICAL FACTORS

The effects of the abnormal mechanical function of the body's parts will be quickly revealed during athletic performance. While structural deviation may not cause difficulty in sedentary individuals, slight deviation may result in severe problems in athletes. Slight structural abnormalities can put extra stress on muscles, tendons, ligaments and bones and result in eventual breakdown of these tissues. Our body's structure is determined by genetics and the environment in which we grow. No matter what many well intentioned, misguided "healers" state, structural deviations *cannot be adjusted or put back into place.* Any suspected anatomical deviation, especially of the spine, must be assessed by a competent sports medicine doctor or sports physiotherapist, as specialised orthopaedic, physiotherapeutic or podiatric management may be indicated. This is of paramount importance in the growing child, as mistakes and poor management during this period may well result in permanent problems.

Heavy training and playing of sport may also result in muscle imbalance situations. Large muscles which are prime movers in locomotion (such as the calf muscles) become over-developed and tight, whereas the opposing muscle (for example, the tibial muscles in shin splints) become relatively weak and subject to stress.

The assessment and treatment of anatomical factors in relation to injury must be left to the sports medicine professionals. This is not an area for the unqualified.

ENVIRONMENTAL FACTORS

Terrain

The ideal playing surface is flat, smooth and resilient. Any variation from this is likely to produce overuse syndromes, secondary to pounding on hard surfaces or compensating for irregular surfaces. When an athlete is running he or she strikes the ground with a force five times that of walking. It does not take much to imagine the considerable repetitive forces transmitted to muscles, bones and joints. Hard surfaces such as hard court tennis courts and dry early season football pitches can increase the impact shock and predispose to the various shin soreness syndromes (p.262). Conversely, wet boggy conditions may increase the likelihood of Achilles tendonitis (p.258) and plantar fasciitis (p.255).

Equipment

Athletic equipment and implements may also have a bearing on overuse injuries. A classical example is the influence of tennis grip size on the incidence of "tennis elbow" (chapter 10).

The major piece of athletic equipment implicated in overuse injuries is the athlete's shoe. There is no all-purpose shoe. The day of the sandshoe which was used for all sports is long gone. One must select the correct shoe for a particular sport; a tennis shoe will not make a jogging shoe.

Any shoe used for athletic pursuits must fit well to avoid friction blisters and skin problems. The shoe must fit adequately in width and length. There is usually a little give in the width of a shoe; therefore a little snugness is allowable, remembering that there should be adequate room in the toe box to prevent crowding of the toes. No give can be achieved in the length of a shoe, as it does not stretch in this direction. When trying new shoes, make sure this is done with the same socks that will be worn when using the particular shoe. It is important to monitor the fit of children's sports shoes frequently, as they can rapidly outgrow their shoes in the course of one season. A detailed description of running shoes is given on page 248.

9
RUNNING INJURIES

There are many thousands of people running and jogging in Australia today and despite the advances in the technology of design and manufacture of running shoes, the average runner will suffer injuries. Runners are a unique group, as they comprise a very healthy segment of the population. They usually have little difficulty in performing other athletic endeavours. Contemporary runners are logging many kilometres which will magnify the deleterious effect of any basic anatomical variance that could be tolerated in most sporting activity. Accumulated impact stress to the lower extremity is found in distance runners.

CAUSES OF INJURY

TRAINING ERRORS

As stated in the introduction to this section on the overuse problem, training errors are the single most common cause of injury. American studies on running injuries have demonstrated that excessive kilometres accounted for 29 per cent of all training errors. Other significant errors are intense workouts, primarily "interval" training, and rapid changes in training programs. Interval training is where there are multiple runs of short duration with little rest in between bursts. This is an anaerobic type of training and if abused, will produce early fatigue in muscles, creating a potential injury situation. These training errors do not let the body recover from cumulative fatigue and microtrauma. This leads to eventual breakdown of the body's soft tissues.

At the present time there is a "mileage mania" and novice runners feel that the more kilometres they log, the better they are able to run. This philosophy is extolled by the popular press, and runners attempt to emulate the published feats of accomplished runners, who thrive on long distances. The way "mileage" is accumulated is extremely important. It must be a slow process allowing the body to adapt to small increases in loads, approximately 10 per cent per week. A good training program should allow for hard-easy days with long distances attempted on only three or four days a week. Runners wishing to achieve marathon status should seek out the clubs or clinics in their city which cater for marathoners, so that the novice can glean information from experienced runners.

ANATOMICAL FACTORS

Biomechanics

To understand the causes of many of the overuse injuries to the lower limb it is necessary to gain an understanding of the mechanics of human motion (*biomechanics*). Biomechanics is a complex and exact science, therefore this book does not delve into its depths. A biomechanical approach to the treatment of injury is to seek out the mechanical reason for breakdown of the body's tissues; correct the fault and stop the injury from re-occurring.

The mechanics of motion can be simplified by following the actions of the "ideal" foot during the phase of running from where the foot strikes the ground to where it leaves the running surface. This phase is termed the stance phase of gait.

To aid the description of the foot during running, two terms must be defined. These are *foot pronation* and *foot supination*.
Pronation   This is the term used to describe the action of the forefoot as it rotates inwards, lowering the arch of the foot.
Supination   This describes the opposite action where the forefoot rotates outwards, raising the arch of the foot away from the ground.

The stance phase of gait can be broken down into three distinct sequences for analysis:
1 foot strike;
2 mid-support;
3 takeoff.
1   *Foot strike*   The part of the foot which first contacts the running surface is normally the outside of the heel. The rest of the foot is then lowered to the ground and the forefoot begins to pronate (roll inwards).
2   *Mid-support*   The forefoot continues to pronate to allow the arch of the foot to act as a shock absorber and adapt the foot to the running surface. As the body weight of the runner moves over the foot, it begins to supinate so that at mid-stance (where

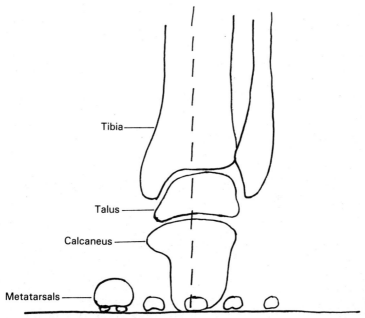

Figure 9.1 The neutral foot.

the body weight lies directly over the foot) the foot will reach a situation where it is completely balanced (not supinated or pronated). This is the ideal situation where all the bones of the foot should line up. It is termed the *neutral position*. Obviously, when the foot is in the neutral position there is a normal arch and the foot is neither pronated (low arch) or supinated (high arch) (fig. 9.1).

The neutral foot (normal arch) is ideal because arch stability is maintained without the muscles and ligaments which support the arch needing to work too hard to control the forefoot against the forces of body weight and gravity. This situation does not place excessive stress on other joints and structures which support body weight. Therefore, it is less likely that the neutral foot will be associated with overuse injuries because the muscles and joint structures are in the "ideal" alignment and are not subjected to excessive stress during locomotion. The non-neutral foot allows for instability and the muscles work out of phase and inefficiently to maintain balance.

3   *Takeoff*   During this phase the foot supinates past the neutral position so that the bones of the foot become locked to form a

rigid lever to transmit the power developed by the leg muscles to push the runner forward.

The Effect of Foot Movements on the Leg

The leg is forced to follow the actions of the foot. When the arch of the foot is lowered (pronated) the shin bone (tibia) rotates inward (fig. 9.2), and when the arch is raised (supinated) the leg rotates outward. This rotation of the shin bone (tibia) has a twisting effect on the knee joint and kneecap and can also influence the mechanics of the hip and lower back.

Overpronating Feet: The Biomechanical Problem

Unfortunately, many athletic feet do not achieve the neutral position during weight bearing. These problem feet tend to pronate excessively, causing the arch of the foot to appear "flat" when weight bearing. American statistics suggest that approximately 40 per cent of runners have the problem of over-pronating feet.

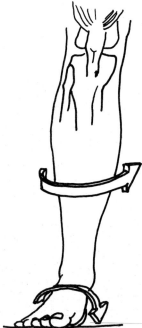

Figure 9.2   The effect of pronation on the limb.

Pronation causes imbalance which leads to fatigue during running and this chronic fatigue leads to abnormal running styles that will eventually develop an overuse injury such as:

- overstretching the ligaments that support the various joints of the foot;
- overworking the muscles that support the arch of the foot;
- causing excessive rotation of the shin bone which may lead to complaints of the knee, hip and lower back.

Anatomical Deviations

Pronating feet are associated with laxity of the supporting ligaments of the foot. These feet appear to have a normal arch when not weight bearing, but flatten out on standing. The overpronated foot is usually a compensation for certain anatomical deviations.

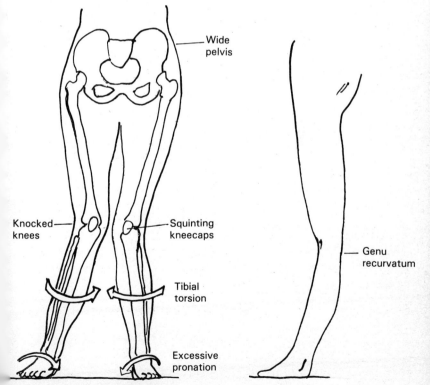

Figure 9.3 Poor alignment.

Knocked knees are usually associated with a backward curving of the leg (genu recurvatum) and small mobile kneecaps which squint inwards. This limb posture will place excessive stress on the inside of the foot causing excessive pronation during running, dancing and jumping. Because of the pronation and its associated overstressing, overuse syndromes are common at the foot, shin and knee. This type of posture is common in pre-adolescent children, especially females, and is often quickly outgrown. If this limb posture persists into adulthood, problems with injury will occur.

The feet in figure 9.4 are often referred to as Morton's feet and are probably traceable to unusual ligament laxity in childhood. The typical flexible forefoot has a big toe which is shorter than the second toe. This situation impairs the effectiveness of the pushoff power of the big toe. The forefoot must roll inwards (pronate) in order for the big toe to make contact with the ground during the propulsion part of the "push off" phase of gait. Besides the many overuse syndromes associated with overpronation, the short great toe may lead to excessive stress on the first toe joint causing the deviation of the great toe (hallux valgus) and the formation of a "bunion" (fig. 9.5).

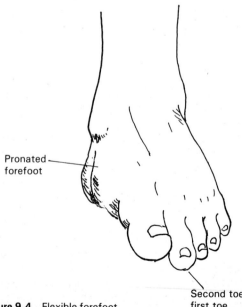

Pronated forefoot

Second toe longer than first toe

Figure 9.4   Flexible forefoot.

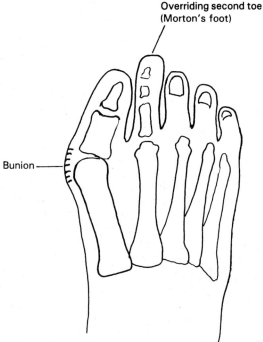

Overriding second toe
(Morton's foot)

Bunion —

Figure 9.5 Hallux valgus (with bunion).

Tight Calf Muscles (Equinus Deformity)

The equinus deformity can be either caused by a congenital abnormality or acquired. Only the acquired problem will be discussed in this book.

The calf muscle complex is comprised of the gastrocnemius muscle, the soleus muscle and the Achilles tendon. These structures tend to become overdeveloped and tight in athletes, as they provide much of the strong propulsive force in locomotion. They tend to overpower the anterior muscles which stabilise the foot and arch. Excessive tightness of the calf muscles will cause prolonged pronation of the forefoot to enable the leg to pass over the foot. During the mid-stance of gait, 10 degrees of ankle dorsiflexion (the motion of the foot moving up towards the leg) are needed for efficient locomotion.

Not all structural problems of the lower limb can be attributed to overpronation. There are many subtleties of limb alignment and

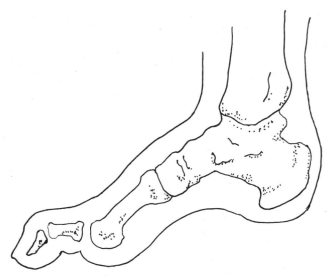

Figure 9.6   The cavus foot.

joint position which may pose problems. One of the most common is the high arched or cavus foot (fig. 9.6).

The high arched foot is stable and not very flexible. Because of its rigidity, it acts as a very poor shock absorber and is often a problem in long distance runners, whereas multi-directional sports and sprinting suit the cavus foot. The poor shock-absorbing capability allows increased shock to be transmitted to the foot, leg, knee and hip predisposing the body to injuries such as stress fractures (p.267) and plantar fasciitis (p. 255).

It is evident from the above discussion that there are two major biomechanical problems in runners. Excessive pronation during the stance phase of gait may produce excessive tortional forces and stress on various joints and soft tissue structures and cause overuse injuries. A rigid high arched foot, which doesn't pronate enough, allows too much impact shock to be transmitted to structures of the foot and leg.

Muscle Imbalance

Long distance runners are very susceptible to strength-flexibility imbalance between muscle groups. The more an athlete runs, the greater the likelihood of the propulsive muscles, namely the calf muscles, the hamstrings and the hip flexors, becoming tight. The tighter the calf muscles become, the more they interfere with the optimal function of the foot and increase the likelihood of excessive foot pronation and its associated problems. A tight hamstring can alter the swing of the leg in running and affect the posture of the pelvis and lower spine and therefore induce poor biomechanics of the foot and leg. Tightness of the hip flexors and back muscles will cause the pelvis to rotate and place stress of the joints of the lower spine and hips.

Conversely, other muscles in runners become weak in relation to the tight muscles. The muscles which attach to the front of the shin (the tibial muscles) become weak and when associated with increased impact shock and poor biomechanics, shin splints (p.262) and tibial stress fracture (p.267) will develop. The quadriceps muscle also may become weaker, especially the medial (inside thigh) muscle which stabilises the kneecap. This will predispose to peripatella stress syndrome (p.270). Weakness can also be found in the abdominal and hip extensors (gluteal muscles) and can compound the forward rotation of the pelvis and its association with low back pain (see "Back, hip and pelvic pain in running athletes", this chapter, p.285).

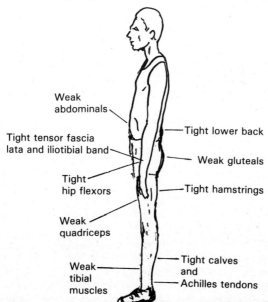

Weak abdominals

Tight tensor fascia lata and iliotibial band

Tight hip flexors

Weak quadriceps

Weak tibial muscles

Tight lower back

Weak gluteals

Tight hamstrings

Tight calves and Achilles tendons

Figure 9.7 Common muscle imbalances which develop in runners.

ENVIRONMENTAL FACTORS

Terrain

Any variation from a flat, smooth running surface is likely to produce an overuse injury as a result of pounding on hard surfaces or compensating for transverse grades, irregular surfaces and hills.

The average road has a drainage slope of 5-10 degrees, depending on the number of resurfacings. Running on a transverse grade increases the pronation of the uphill foot which may place stress on structures such as the plantar fascia, tibial muscles and the knee. On the downhill foot there is increased impact on the outside of the foot and this may cause stress fractures of the bones of the foot.

Running uphill will increase the tension on the plantar fascia, especially if the calf muscles are tight. Downhill running places increased tension on the knee mechanisms as they contract to decelerate the body. This can accentuate knee problems, particularly of the kneecap.

The Running Shoe

Most long distance running is done on hard surfaces which provide little shock-absorbing capacity. Forces two to three times body weight occur at foot strike and runners should run on relatively soft surfaces such as a grassy footpath or soft road shoulder. Since this is almost never practical, the next best alternative is to wear an adequately constructed shoe that will provide protection for the lower extremity.

Jogger-type shoes account for nearly 30-40 per cent of all sports shoes sold. A large proportion of these are the cheap imitation running shoes, marketed through the chain outlets. Some medical authorities in the United States have stated that the chance of injury wearing these cheap shoes when running is approximately 80 per cent. These shoes are fine for casual or school wear, but are a disaster for the serious recreational or competitive runner. During the past few years, there has been a revolution in the design and number of brands of running shoes and selection is fraught with confusion. Certain brands and models may be ideal for one athlete because of his or her foot shape and style and problematic for another. Guidance on shoe selection should be sought from a reputable shoe retailer who deals with runners and their problems, a sports podiatrist and by consulting the popular

running press for their current shoe evaluations. Factors that should be taken into consideration include:
- foot shape (pronated or high arched);
- foot flexibility (flexible or rigid forefoot);
- distance run;
- running style;
- fit and comfort.

Regardless of the manufacturer and model, there are certain criteria which the athlete should look for in a running shoe. A good training shoe should provide cushioning, support and stability, yet it must maintain a reasonable degree of flexibility and lightness. The outer sole should be of a carbon rubber construction in a studded or "waffle" design, as this type of sole provides traction and stability. Flexibility of the sole is important, especially at the level of the toe joints to allow bending during the "toe off" phase of gait. Construction of the mid-sole must be of a material designed for maximum shock absorption and have a "short memory" after compression so that it can reform in preparation for the next foot strike. The heel should be raised 12-18 mm to allow for additional shock and to take the stress off the calf muscles.

The heel counter should be firm to control the hind foot and prevent shoe distortion. A well moulded Achilles pad is essential to prevent irritation and blistering. A round toe box with adequate height is important to prevent toe crowding. Outside, nylon mesh reinforced with suede on the toe box and heel counter is probably the best construction. Nylon mesh allows the foot to breathe and

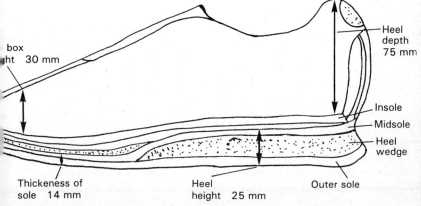

Figure 9.8 The anatomy of the running shoe.

Table 9.1   Summary of factors associated with runner's overuse injury.

Training errors	1	Too much — too soon
	2	Overtraining
	3	Too great a distance
Anatomical factors	1	Biomechanical faults
		(a) malalignment of the limb and compensatory pronation
		(b) Pes cavus
	2	Muscle strength-flexibility imbalance
Environmental factors	1	Terrain
		(a) Surface and impact shock
		(b) Road slope
		(c) Hill running
	2	Shoe design and wear.

dry quickly and allows for easy laundering of the shoe. Weight of a good training shoe should be approximately 300 to 350 grams (fig. 9.8).

THE APPROACH TO THE TREATMENT OF RUNNING INJURIES

Many a distance runner has had his or her career ended by the injudicious treatment of a running injury. Immobilisation, prolonged rest, surgery and repeated cortisone injections have the potential to end permanently a career and are virtually never indicated in the treatment of running injuries. The treatment plan consists of finding and correcting the cause of injury, providing symptomatic relief, the supervision of the athlete's rehabilitation until he or she has regained the former level of training, and instigating a prevention program.

SYMPTOMATIC RELIEF

I.C.E. (ice, compression and elevation)

This is the first aid regime of choice. The rationale for its use and the methods of application are well illustrated in the section of the book covering rehabilitation (chapter 5). Physiotherapy modalities and anti-inflammatory drugs are often needed in the very painful or refractory injury.

Rest

Total rest is undoubtedly the most unacceptable form of treatment for a runner, therefore a reduction in training distance is more appropriate. The training routine is altered to provide a level of activity devoid of pain: any action that brings on discomfort *must be stopped*. However, at times, total rest of a limb may be essential, the duration depending on the severity or chronic recurrence of the injury. During this period of rest, other forms of exercise such as swimming and cycling must be undertaken to maintain cardiovascular fitness.

A very common mistake following a period of rest is returning to vigorous training once pain-free, only to have the injury recur. A gradual return to training must be undertaken to allow the damaged part to develop its specific strength and endurance and for the runner to regain an appropriate level of cardiovascular endurance.

REHABILITATION

As stated repeatedly throughout this book, exercise is the most important modality in the promotion of healing, the restoration of function and an early return to sport. Athletes must realise the importance of regaining full strength and flexibility and not depend merely on a "magic box of tricks". Ice and other modalities should be considered as adjuncts, providing muscle relaxation, pain relief and the reduction of swelling.

CORRECTION OF THE CAUSE OF INJURY

The correction of training faults and the alteration of the terrain the athlete runs over were discussed previously. A common sense approach to running will alleviate these problems.

Excessive wear and distortion of the shoe can predispose an athlete to injury. A shoe should be placed on a table and viewed from behind. The heel counter should be perpendicular to the ground. Any distortion, especially towards the inside, will render the shoe useless for running. Always check new shoes before purchasing for any distortion due to faulty manufacture (fig. 9.9).

Another common problem with shoes is allowing the outer edge of the new sole to wear down creating instability across the heel during foot strike. This area should be filled with a suitable

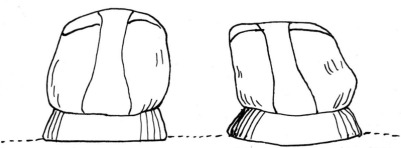

Figure 9.9 Distortion of a shoe due to excessive pronation — rear view, right foot pronated.

preparation (for example, Shoe Goo) to build the shoe up to normal height. Care must be taken not to build this area up above the height of the rest of the sole, as an increase in height will force the foot into pronation and cause further injury.

The diagnosis and correction of anatomical factors require the attention of the relevant profession. Muscle imbalance and the relationship of posture and movement to injury are in the realm of the sports physiotherapist. Major anatomical deviations and gross or persistant injury may require the management of sports medicine doctors or orthopaedic surgeons.

Earlier in this chapter under the section on "Biomechanics", the role of foot pronation in running was discussed (p.242). Many studies have shown that excessive pronation is one of the major causes of foot and leg problems in runners. As discussed previously, certain anatomical deviations, such as the poor alignment syndrome, flexible forefoot and tight calf muscles, are all compensated for by excessive pronation. The correction of this excessive pronation can be achieved by a special appliance called an "orthotic".

Orthotics

An orthotic appliance is a specially built insert placed between the foot and the sole of the shoe to position the foot near the neutral position (p.241). The rationale for its use is to allow the foot to function as near as possible about the neutral position (fig. 9.1) so that excessive pronation of the foot will be reduced, removing the abnormal stresses placed on the foot and lower limb when running (fig. 9.10).

Scientific evidence collected in the USA has shown that when using an orthotic, where indicated, a smoother running form is

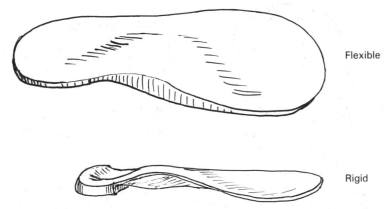

Flexible

Rigid

Figure 9.10 Orthotics.

achieved with decreased impact shock, a more efficient use of muscles and more even shoe wear. A perfectly balanced foot decreases the likelihood of an overuse injury.

An orthotic is not a simple arch support. It is a special device that is moulded from a plaster cast of the foot which has been placed in the neutral position. A sports podiatrist with special skills and equipment should be consulted to dispense properly and fine tune the appliance. Orthotics are not a panacea for the treatment of all running injuries. Often the selection of a better running shoe may achieve the same result.

THE PREVENTION OF RUNNING INJURIES

A Realistic Training Program

The training schedule must:
- cater for adequate rest and recuperation;
- have achievable goals; a marathon cannot be achieved with only a few months of training, for example;
- make increments of load that will not induce injury. A practical rule of thumb is an increase of approximately 10 per cent per week.

Shoe Maintenance

Abnormal wear of the sole should be countered with products such as Shoe Goo. Make regular checks for excessive distortion and wear of the heel counter. The mid-sole should also be checked to ensure it has not lost its shock-absorbing capacity.

A Proper Warm-up and an Ongoing Strength/Flexibility Program

For warm-up details see chapter 1. Specific strength-flexibility guidelines for runners are shown in figure 9.11.

Stretch   *Strengthen*

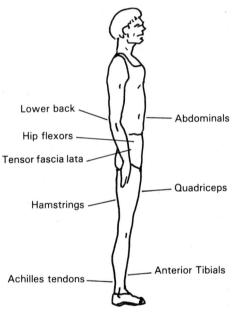

Figure 9.11   Flexibility-strength guide for runners.

SPECIFIC INJURIES COMMON TO RUNNERS

No attempt is made in this book to discuss all the varieties of overuse injuries of the lower leg. Selected syndromes will be presented because of their frequency of incidence in runners.

PLANTAR FASCIITIS

Anatomy

The plantar fascia is a sheath-like structure running from the heel bone (calcaneus) to the base of the toes (fig. 9.12). Its function is to provide strong support for the arch of the foot.

Middle-aged runners are prone to this injury as they develop areas of degeneration, especially at the area where the fascia attaches to the inside of the heel. Excessive force or repetitive stress may then damage the weakened area. This injury is often mistakenly called "heel spur" because a bony spur projecting from the calcaneum is often seen on X-ray. This spur signifies a bony response to chronic inflammation and indicates degenerative

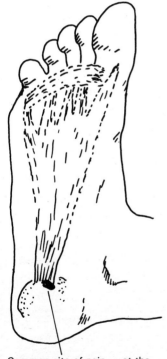

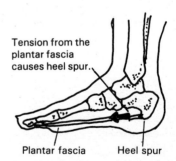

Tension from the plantar fascia causes heel spur.

Plantar fascia   Heel spur

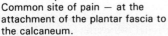

Common site of pain — at the attachment of the plantar fascia to the calcaneum.

Figure 9.12   The plantar fascia.

changes in the area. The heel spur is not a cause of plantar fasciitis, but is a result of the condition.

Cause of Injury

Acute injuries may occur, such as stepping into a hole, or alighting awkwardly onto the edge of a footpath. These injuries result in minor tears to the fascia and, if not properly managed, may develop into a chronic inflammatory condition.

More commonly the injury to the plantar fascia is of the overuse variety. These injuries result from a combination of training errors, anatomical factors and environmental factors. These have been discussed previously and only relevant factors will be discussed here.

The biomechanical problems of excessive pronation (p.242) and the cavus foot (p.246) are implicated in many cases of plantar fasciitis. Excessive pronation causes the arch to over-flatten during weight bearing which places excessive tension on the fascia as it attempts to support the arch. Conversely, the cavus foot because of its rigidity and poor shock-absorbing ability, can also overstress the plantar fascia.

A tight calf muscle group can also pose problems. The tight calf will limit ankle dorsiflexion, which increases the tension on the plantar fascia. Tension is also placed on the fascia with uphill running and on the uphill foot when running across a slope.

Each of the above factors or a combination can cause chronic irritation resulting in microtrauma and the necessary repair process to the attachment of the plantar fascia to the heel bone.

Signs and Symptoms

Pain is usually felt at the back of the arch of the foot. Point tenderness can often be elicited at the attachment site of the plantar fascia to the calcaneum (fig. 6.12). The pain and stiffness is usually most noticeable with the first few steps of the morning, but then abates during the day only to return during or after exercise. This condition is mainly characterised by a slow onset which allows the athlete to run for weeks or even months before seeking attention.

Treatment

This provides mainly symptomatic relief, allowing the condition to heal and correcting the underlying fault. I.C.E. is the first aid

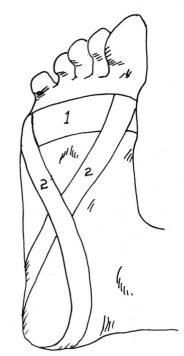

1 Anchor
2 Support for arch
3 Over no. 2
4 Over no. 1 for
   final anchor

Figure 9.13   Taping of the arch of the foot.

modality of choice. A heel doughnut made of felt often relieves pressure over the tender spot. If the runner wishes to continue training, low dye taping of the arch may relieve the strain on the plantar fascia (fig. 9.13).

Physiotherapy management involves the application of selected electromedical modalities to give symptomatic relief and initiating the appropriate stretching exercises for the calf muscles and arch (fig. 1.3(g)). Podiatry assessment and orthotic management may be necessary if biomechanical faults such as excessive pronation or a rigid cavus foot exist. In refractory cases, a local injection of anti-inflammatory steroids into the point of maximum tenderness may be necessary to interrupt the pain cycle. This is usually an extreme measure and one must be mindful of the precautions discussed earlier in this book.

Rehabilitative exercises to maintain the strength and endurance of other muscle groups and joints should be instigated. Activities such as bicycling, swimming or rowing should be encouraged to maintain cardiovascular endurance.

ACHILLES TENDONITIS

This injury is one of the most frequent and disabling in athletics. It is a stress injury to the large tendon which connects the calf muscle to the heel (fig. 9.14).

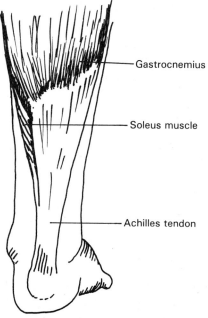

Gastrocnemius

Soleus muscle

Achilles tendon

Figure 9.14   The Achilles tendon (refer also to the section on the calf muscle, chapter 7, p.154).

Cause of Injury

It is thought that either overtraining, biomechanical mal-alignment, lack of adequate heel protection or excessive uphill running may place excessive stress on the tendon. This situation will lead to inflammation and microtrauma to the soft tissues surrounding the tendon, or to microscopic tears within the tendon itself. Achilles tendonitis is often associated with excessive pronation (fig. 9.2) which places excessive stress on the Achilles tendon as the body moves over the weight-bearing foot. The cavus foot (Fig. 9.6) and tight calf muscles also overstress the Achilles during running.

Signs and Symptoms

In the acute phase, the athlete complains of pain and swelling along the tendon. Pain is produced on running and climbing stairs, but infrequently on walking. With the appropriate treatment the acute injury will settle quickly.

Chronic tendonitis is a condition in which the symptoms have been present for many months and would suggest that repetitive microtrauma has caused degeneration within the tendon. Chronic tendonitis poses problems for the athlete as tendons have a poor blood supply; therefore, their rate of healing is very slow (see chapter 2 "Healing of special tissues"). These injuries will eventually heal, but will take many months of dedicated work to achieve results.

Treatment

Initial treatment is rest from pain and an effective I.C.E. regime. A heel pad placed in the shoe may help to reduce tension on the tendon (fig. 7.23). Running should be restricted to within pain-free limits. Extensive physiotherapy and anti-inflammatory medication are usually needed for severe cases.

Rehabilitation includes gentle calf muscle and Achilles stretches (fig.1.3(g)) and toe raises, as described previously in figure 7.21. Isokinetic strengthening is the most suitable form of exercise. Podiatric assessment and orthotic control are often required to prevent re-occurrence. Maintenance exercises for muscular strength and endurance for the other parts of the body as well as bicycling and swimming for cardiovascular endurance must be initiated.

OTHER COMMON FORMS OF ARCH AND FOOT PAIN

Cuboid Syndrome

This syndrome is often confused with plantar fasciitis. However, the pain differs in that it is more prevalent along the lateral side of the foot, whereas plantar fasciitis usually occurs on the inside of the arch. The injury appears to be a locking of the cuboid bone which disturbs its normal range of motion.

Cause of Injury

Symptoms usually appear after the athlete does something to which he or she is unaccustomed. Increasing a training load,

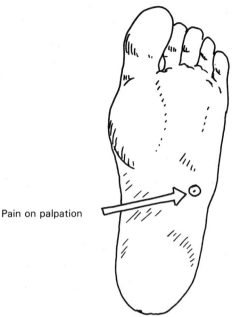

Pain on palpation

Figure 9.15 The cuboid bone and the point of tenderness elicited with the clinician's thumb.

running faster or over uneven terrain, changing surfaces or twisting the foot by tripping can all cause cuboid syndrome. Most patients seen with this problem have pronated feet which allow greater mechanical forces to be applied to the cuboid bone by the outside muscles of the leg (peroneus longus muscle).

Treatment

The most effective management is specific manipulation of the cuboid bone. This technique must be carried out by a competent clinician and I.C.E. and an effective rehabilitation program must follow the manipulative treatment. Recovery time depends on how long the symptoms have been apparent before the patient sought effective treatment.

In the acute phase, low dye strapping (fig. 9.13) can be applied to protect the cuboid bone, especially between manipulative treatments. If excessive pronation is apparent, orthotic control may be indicated.

Interdigital Neuroma

Compression and irritation of the small nerve bundle between the metatarsal bones of the foot can lead to the formation of a neuroma. A neuroma is a small tumor of the nerve bundle (fig. 9.16).

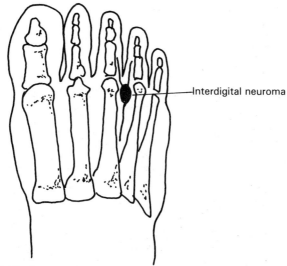

Figure 9.16 Interdigital neuroma — common between the third and fourth metatarsal heads.

Cause of Injury

There has usually been a rapid increase in training load resulting in an insidious onset of pain in the forefoot. The irritating compressive forces which develop the neuroma are often seen in the overpronating foot which allows excessive mobility in the forefoot.

Signs and Symptoms

The point of maximum tenderness is usually between the third and fourth toes. Pain will increase with activity and can spread down the toes. Relief is often achieved by removing the shoe. Once the condition becomes chronic, sensation changes may become apparent along the inside of the toes.

Treatment

Symptomatic relief can be achieved by the reduction of training and the application of I.C.E. Physiotherapy modalities such as ultrasound may help to reduce the inflammatory process. A metatarsal bar may also be placed in the shoe to help relieve pressure on the nerve. If these methods do not produce satisfactory results, a doctor may consider a local anaesthetic and a steroid injection. Most resistant cases require the surgical removal of the inflamed nerve. Orthotic control is necessary in most cases to control the excessive pronation.

SHIN PAIN

There are many causes of chronic leg pain in athletes. Such conditions include muscle hernia, bone tumor, osteomyelitis, muscle strains, inflammation at various sites, circulatory constriction (compartment syndrome), referred pain from the low back, and so on. Because of the vast number of potential causes of pain, any pains that do not settle quickly with an I.C.E. and reduced activity regime must be seen by a sports physician for an accurate diagnosis. In this book the three most common causes of shin pain will be discussed, namely: shin "soreness", "shin splints" and "stress fracture".

Shin Soreness

This is a term used to describe a muscular overuse. It is common in athletes beginning a training program after a layoff, for example, footballers undergoing pre-season training. This condition can affect any of the muscle groups of the lower leg, including the calf muscles.

Heavy training sessions may cause microtrauma to the muscle of the leg. This leads to minor breakdown of muscle tissue and inflammation. I.C.E., stretching and a graduated return to full training should alleviate the symptoms within 72 hours. If the athlete continues to run through the pain, shin soreness may progress into one of the more serious syndromes such as "shin splints".

Shin Splints

"Shin splints" is a lay term which has become a wastebasket category to describe shin pain of any source. The authors suggest

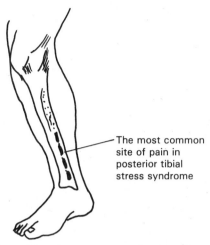

The most common site of pain in posterior tibial stress syndrome

Figure 9.17   The position of tenderness in "shin splints".

that "posterior tibial stress syndrome" is a better term to describe pain on the medial (inside) border of the shin bone (tibia) (fig. 9.17).

Anatomy

There are three muscles (flexor digitorum longus, flexor hallucis longus and tibialis posterior) which anchor onto the inside shaft of the tibia and insert into various positions of the foot and toes (fig. 9.18). Collectively, their function is to stabilise the arch of the foot during the stance phase of gait. Therefore, their role is to counter the pronation forces flattening the arch as the body's weight passes over the foot. The injury described as "shin splints" is fatigue microtrauma to the above muscle tendons where they attach to the shin bone.

Cause of Injury

Control of the foot during running requires a balanced interplay of the muscles of the leg and foot, especially in stabilising the arch. This delicate balance may be disrupted by the overloading of training stress. This overload causes muscle fatigue and the loss of efficiency in shock absorption. Continued physical activity leads to structural stress on the muscle tendon insertion onto the bone with resultant pain and inflammation. This pain leads to

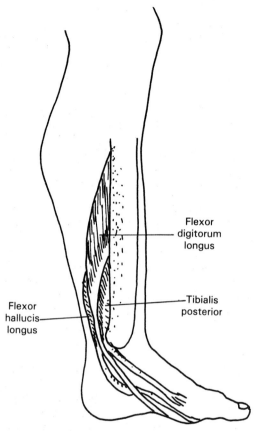

Flexor
digitorum
longus

Flexor
hallucis
longus

Tibialis
posterior

Figure 9.18 The posterior tibial muscles.

involuntary rest of the muscle system and muscle weakness
follows.

Precipitating events include: overuse early in a training
program, a change in running surface or footwear, poor
biomechanics of running due to excessive pronation. As stated
previously, the posterior tibial muscles support the arch during
weight bearing; therefore, excessive pronation will increase the
workload of these muscles, causing their eventual breakdown.
Muscle imbalance can also play a role in the development of "shin
splints". The calf muscles become very tight and overdeveloped
with running sports, disturbing the fine balance with the posterior
tibial muscles, and causing fatigue in them. "Posterior tibial stress
syndrome" is mostly seen in the less well conditioned athlete, early

in a season, or with athletes unaware of the importance of stretching and gradual conditioning.

Signs and Symptoms

Symptoms begin with mild to moderate discomfort over the posterior lower shaft of the tibia, with or without localised swelling (fig. 9.17). In the early phase, rest from activity will relieve pain. However, with continued training the pain will become more prominent and long lasting until pain is experienced at rest. Most sufferers of shin splints will show marked impairment, one-legged hopping on the affected side, due to both pain and weakness.

Treatment

The initial aims are to control pain and reduce inflammation and swelling through I.C.E., anti-inflammatory medication, reduced activity/rest and physiotherapy.

Reduced activity/rest is essential to resolve the problem early. If running and training are not reduced to totally pain-free limits, the injury will not heal. Because this injury involves the tendinous portion of the muscle where it anchors to the bone, healing can be a slow, arduous process, especially if pain and discomfort are long standing. The reasons are that tendinous/bony insertion injury has an extended healing time because of the poor blood supply to tendon tissue and if the injury has been allowed to become chronic, the added complication is a weak immature scar.

Physiotherapy management involves modalities to increase circulation and promote healing, as well as starting the appropriate rehabilitative stretching and strengthening exercises. As described above, muscle imbalance is a common finding in "shin splint" patients. The tight, overdeveloped calf muscles must be placed through a comprehensive stretching program to increase their length and reduce the pronation forces applied to the forefoot during weight bearing. Relevant stretches are depicted in figure 1.3(g).

To gain a strong, mature scar in the damaged muscles and to return these muscles to their full strength, power and endurance, a comprehensive retraining program must be prescribed. In the physiotherapy gymnasium equipment such as the Cybex, Orthotron or Rotagym are used with exercise protocols to redevelop the parameters of strength, power and endurance.

Rehabilitation without the sophisticated isokinetic and variable

a. Picking up marbles with the toes.

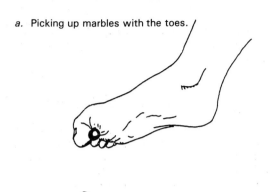

b. Using surgical rubber.

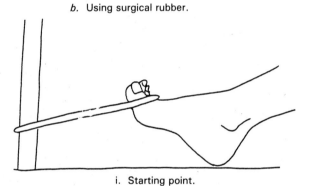

i. Starting point.

Dorsiflexion and inversion

ii. Pull the ankle up and in.

Figure 9.19 Strengthening exercises for the posterior tibial muscles.

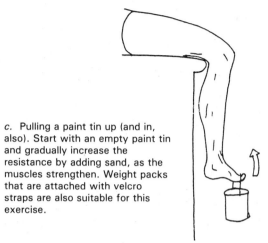

c. Pulling a paint tin up (and in, also). Start with an empty paint tin and gradually increase the resistance by adding sand, as the muscles strengthen. Weight packs that are attached with velcro straps are also suitable for this exercise.

Figure 9.19 Strengthening exercises (continued).

resistance used in the physiotherapy rooms involves the simple strengthening exercises depicted in figure 9.19. Alternate cardiovascular training programs must be set for the athlete to maintain fitness. A simple test that can be used to determine whether an athlete can resume light training is to make the athlete attempt one-legged jumps (hops) on the affected leg. If he or she can complete 20 or so repetitions without pain, light training can be resumed. Taping the arch of the foot (fig. 9.13) may help reduce the stress to the posterior tibial muscles in this early stage.

STRESS FRACTURE

A stress fracture is a partial crack in the hard outer casing of the bone as a result of non-violent stress that is applied in a rhythmic, repeated, sub-threshold manner. The excessive forces applied to the bone provide a signal for it to "remodel" and lay down extra bone to withstand the stress. The first step in "remodelling" is for cells called osteoclasts to remove bone actively. At this stage symptoms develop as the formation of new bone lags behind. This discrepancy between the removal of bone and new bone formation means the area is weakened and susceptible to fracture. If the stress to the bone is removed by adequate rest the remodelling process can be completed and the stress fracture will heal.

The most common site of stress fracture in athletes is along the inside shaft of the tibia (shin bone). Fractures are also common to the outside leg bone (the fibular) and to the long bones of the foot. The authors believe that most stress fractures are the end-stage of untreated overuse syndromes, such as posterior tibial stress syndrome and plantar fasciitis. That is, if these syndromes are left untreated and the athlete continues to attempt to run through pain for many weeks, he or she will develop stress fractures as a result of the initial soft tissue damage and muscle fatigue exposing the bone to undue stress.

Causes of Stress Fractures

Continuous heavy training will cause muscle fatigue and therefore increase stress on the bone which will then attempt to remodel. Other factors, such as a change in running surface, use of poor quality running shoes or muscle imbalance, may cause a stress fracture. From our clinical experience, a biomechanical problem in conjunction with training overload appears to be the primary cause (fig. 9.20).

Excessive pronation flattens the arch, increasing forces on the bones of the foot and via the leg muscles acting on the arch;

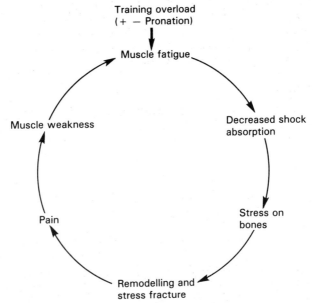

Figure 9.20   Causes of stress fracture.

increased stress is also applied to the long bones of the leg. Excessive pronation is not the only biomechanical problem implicated in stress fractures. A cavus foot (fig. 9.6) is often very rigid and has poor shock-absorbing capacity.

Females seem to be very susceptible to stress/overuse problems. This is because many females have a limb posture that consists of a wide pelvis, inward slanting thighs, and knocked knees, which also curve backwards (fig. 9.3). The poor alignment and biomechanics that this posture creates can cause early muscle fatigue so that more stress is absorbed by the bones that normally lead to a higher incidence of stress fracture.

Signs and Symptoms

There is usually a gradual onset of pain in the area of the fracture during activity. This pain is relieved with rest. If the athlete persists in training, pain will start at the same time as the activity and is often not relieved with rest. Local swelling may occur, particularly after activity.

X-rays taken in the early stages usually do not show a stress fracture. Four to eight weeks after the onset of pain the healing bone (callus) may be visible if the appropriate treatment has been carried out. Therefore, a clear X-ray of the painful area does not rule out the diagnosis of stress fracture. However, a specialised X-ray technique called the nuclear bone scan can detect stress fractures in the early stage of development.

Treatment

The treatment plan is the same as applied to any overuse syndrome. The principles are:
1 Rest from running until the fractures heal and the pain subsides, usually four to six weeks minimum.
2 Provide symptomatic relief with I.C.E., physiotherapy and medication.
3 Begin the appropriate rehabilitative stretching and strengthening exercises for the muscle groups involved.
4 Employ orthotic control if indicated.
5 Maintain cardiovascular fitness with swimming and/or cycling.
6 When asymptomatic, there must be a slow, gradual return to sport. If too fast a return is attempted, the symptoms will re-occur quickly.

KNEE PAIN IN RUNNERS

"Runner's knee" is a non-specific term describing knee pain with a variety of signs, symptoms and diagnoses. The most common-sense way to approach knee pain in athletes is by the anatomical location of the symptoms, for example, around the kneecap (peripatella), medial, lateral or within the joint structures (intra-articular). Major causes of knee pain are listed in table 9.2. Because of the complexity of athletic knee pain, it must be stressed that precise diagnosis must be left to the experienced clinician who has an understanding of the mechanics and pathology of athletic injury.

Table 9.2   Major causes of knee pain.

Peripatella	*Lateral*
Patella tendonitis	Iliotibial band friction syndrome
Quadriceps tendonitis	Bursitis
Subluxing or dislocating patella	Popliteus tendonitis
Osgood-Schlatter's disease	Biceps femoris tendonitis
Prepatella bursitis	
Peripatella stress	
Chondromalacia patellae	
Medial	*Intraarticular*
Pes anserine bursitis	Torn medial meniscus
Voschel's bursitis	Discoid meniscus
Stress fracture, proximal tibia	Cystic, or degenerative meniscus
	Collateral or cruciate ligament tears
	Osteochondral fracture
	Loose bodies
	Synovial plica

It is not within the scope of this book to review all of the conditions of the knee shown in table 9.2. Consequently, the authors have selected for discussion the two most common overuse syndromes of the knee that they see in practice. These are "peripatellar stress syndrome" and "iliotibial band friction syndrome".

Peripatellar Stress Syndrome

This condition describes symptoms arising from the soft tissues that stabilise the kneecap (patella) in its sliding joint with the thigh bone (femur). This joint is called the patello-femoral joint (fig. 9.21). Recent studies and the authors' experience indicate that pain

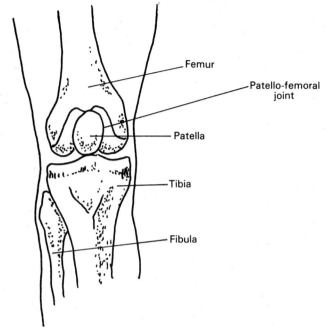

Figure 9.21 The patello-femoral joint (from in front).

around the kneecap is the most common knee symptom in athletes.

Often pain arising from the patello-femoral joint is given the diagnosis of "chondromalacia patellae". This term is used to describe destruction of smooth articular lining on the under surface of the kneecap and diagnosis is made from X-rays and other tests. Thus, the term "chondromalacia patellae" should be reserved for gross pathological changes of the articular cartilage such as in osteoarthritis. Chondromalacia can result from direct trauma such as motor vehicle accidents and dislocation of the patella. It is often present with congenital abnormalities such as bipartite patellae. It is also seen in patello-femoral gross malalignment common in some adolescent females.

The destruction of articular cartilage is rare in the fit, healthy athletic population. The authors believe that labelling athletically induced kneecap pain as "chondromalacia patellae" is inappropriate. Therefore, the term "peripatellar stress syndrome" should be used to label pain arising in the soft tissues supporting the patello-femoral joint. This term is also preferable to the lay term of "runner's knee".

Anatomy

The structures that control the patello-femoral joint can be dynamic or static. Dynamic structures are the muscles that exert pull on the patello-femoral joint via their attachments. The primary muscle action is by the quadriceps muscles through the quadriceps tendon during extension of the knee. The vastus medialis oblique (VMO) plays an important role in stabilising the patella against its tendency to drift laterally. Dynamic lateral force is applied to the patella via the vastus lateralis muscle and a slip of the iliotibial band.

Static structures which exert control on the patella are the patellar ligament, the capsule and its various thickened bands

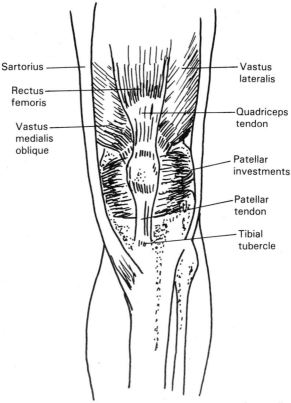

Figure 9.22 Dynamic and static structures which support the patello-femoral joint.

(retinacula). Collectively, these structures can be termed the "patella investments" which support the kneecap against displacement.

Below the quadriceps tendon is a fluid-filled sac, the suprapatellar bursa. The term "bursitis" is used to describe inflammation and swelling of a bursa. The patellar tendon sits below the patella and joins onto the shin bone (tibia). A stress injury to this tendon with resultant tendonitis is labelled "jumper's knee". Figure 9.22 illustrates all structures, both dynamic and static, that support the patello-femoral joint.

Cause of Injury

As with all overuse problems the precipitating events include alteration of training programs, changing running surfaces, footwear faults, and biomechanical and anatomical problems. Most of these situations are covered in depth throughout this section on running injuries. However, the biomechanical and anatomical factors need special attention, as the authors believe that they are the frequent cause of injury to the patella.

During running, the knee must flex and extend; consequently the patella must slide up and down in the groove of the femur, the so-called patello-femoral joint (fig. 9.21). Problems arise when the patella is forced to track incorrectly in this groove.

Anatomical alignment can have great bearing on the tracking of the kneecap. A high riding patella (patella alta) which "squints" inwards is unstable and has a tendency to stress the patella investments and is often prone to subluxation or dislocation. The location of the point where the patellar tendon inserts onto the tibia is an important factor in the tracking mechanism. A more laterally placed tibial tubercle leads to poor tracking of the patella towards the outside. A simple measure of this tracking mechanism is the "Q" angle described in figure 9.23. The average "Q" angle in men is 14 degrees and females 17 degrees.

Females with a wide pelvis, and knocked knees (genu valgum) curved backwards (genu recurvatum), the "poor alignment syndrome" (p.243), have a more laterally placed tibial tubercle and a "Q" angle greater than 17 degrees. Malrotation of the tibia such as excessive external rotation can also lead to greater "Q" angles and poor tracking.

The presence of mechanical problems within the knee itself can lead to patello-femoral pain. For example, with gross instability due to collateral or cruciate ligament laxity (chapter 7, "Joint

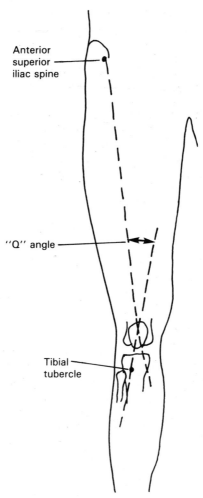

Anterior superior iliac spine

"Q" angle

Tibial tubercle

Figure 9.23 The ''Q'' angle. The ''Q'' angle is the angle between: (a) a line from the anterior superior iliac spine through the midpoint of the patella (representing the pull of the quadriceps) and (b) a line from the tibial tubercle through the midpoint of the patella with the knee fully extended.

injuries''), a torn meniscus or loose bodies can place extra strain on the quadriceps mechanism to stabilise the knee joint structures, eventually causing pain.

In runners, the major biomechanical problem in poor tracking of the patella is excessive pronation, described previously in this

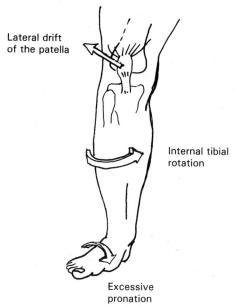

Lateral drift
of the patella

Internal tibial
rotation

Excessive
pronation

Figure 9.24 Excessive pronation of the foot producing lateral drift of the patella.

section (p.242). Overpronation of the foot during weight bearing will cause excessive internal rotation of the tibia, therefore forcing the patella to drift and track more laterally towards the outside of the knee (fig. 9.24).

The poor tracking of the patella will cause stress to the soft tissues which stabilise the patella in its groove, resulting in breakdown of these tissues, followed by inflammation and repair by scar tissue. If the lateral drift of the patella is great, the undersurface of the patella may impinge on the outer lip of the femoral groove (fig. 9.25).

Muscle imbalance can also play a role in the lateral drift of the patella. The quadriceps muscles insert via the quadriceps and patella tendons onto the tibia. The action of the quadriceps muscles is to straighten the knee and, in doing so, pull the patella through the groove in the femur. Because the bulk of the quadriceps lie on the outside of the thigh, the tendency is for the patella to be pulled laterally. To counter this tendency of the patella to drift to the outside, one of the muscles of the quadriceps group, vastus medialis oblique (VMO), attaches to the outside

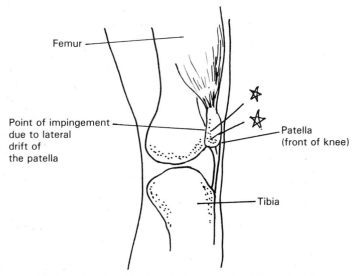

Figure 9.25   Impingement of the patella on the lateral femoral groove.

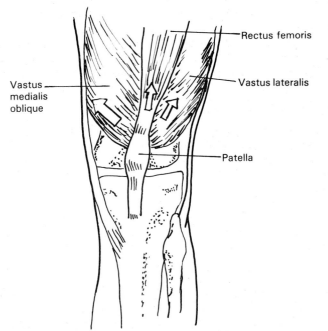

Figure 9.26   Vastus medialis oblique stabilises the patella against lateral drift.

of the patella to hold it in the femoral groove during movements of the knee (fig. 9.26).

Poor tracking of the patella, injury to the quadriceps muscles of the knee joint, or poor rehabilitation following surgery or injury will result in wastage and weakening of the quadriceps, especially the VMO. A weak VMO will also cause extensive drift of the patella and a resultant peripatellar stress syndrome (fig. 9.27).

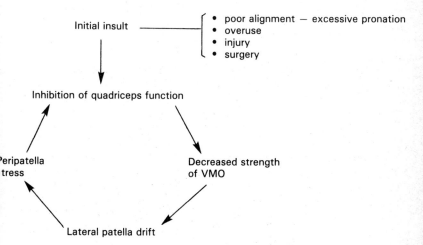

Figure 9.27   The quadriceps muscle imbalance quandary.

Signs and Symptoms

The chief symptom is pain felt around the knee during physical activity. Classically, this pain is pronounced when climbing stairs, or running hills, or doing deep knee bends and squats. Swelling of the knee is often evident and "clicking" (crepitus) may be experienced under the kneecap. The knee joint often feels weak and can give way or lock in various positions. A history of so-called giving way, locking and localised swelling may give the impression that the injury is of knee cartilage origin (chapter 7, "Joint injuries"). Diagnostic skill and specialised techniques such as X-rays and arthroscopic examination are often necessary to eliminate the idea of cartilage (meniscus) injury.

Often patients complain of feeling something go out and back into place within the knee at the time of injury. This situation usually indicates a pronounced lateral shift of the kneecap which leads to partial dislocation (subluxation) of the kneecap. Young adolescent females are prone to this injury, especially with poor alignment (fig. 9.3). Most of these patients respond to conservative treatment; severe cases may need orthopaedic surgery.

Treatment

The initial step is to provide symptomatic relief and inhibit the inflammatory process. Control of symptoms is primarily achieved by activity modification. Sports participation must be within pain-free limits. Pain producing activities such as hill running or jumping must be eliminated. An I.C.E. regime must be stringently maintained to reduce pain and associated symptoms. With severe pain and swelling, physiotherapy modalities and anti-inflammatory medications are indicated. The rehabilitation of a knee joint injury is complex. It takes clinical experience and training to select the appropriate strengthening and stretching exercises, plus the level of resistance and repetitions to be applied. A definitive treatment plan is not the aim of this book; however, some simple practical guidelines will be discussed.

A progressive strengthening program must be initiated as soon as possible. Any knee joint pathology, whether it be a direct injury or overuse, will cause a progressive weakening and wastage of the quadriceps muscles, especially the vastus medialis oblique (VMO). This progressive deterioration in the VMO will lead to the quadriceps muscle quandary depicted in figure 9.27.

Initial quadriceps exercises should involve the straight leg raise technique with the weighted boot (fig. 7.2). Because discomfort and strain often develop in the upper thigh (hip flexors) when the resistance reaches 6 to 8 kilograms, the technique should then be shifted to knee extension exercises.

Traditionally, knee extension exercise for quadriceps rehabilitation has been done from 90 degrees of flexion (fig. 7.3). Recent studies have shown that this technique, while improving muscle strength, risks further damage to the smooth sliding surfaces of the patello-femoral joint. The compromise is to use a lifting technique from 15 degrees of knee flexion (fig. 7.36).

Not only is this technique safer than the lifting through a full range by reducing stress on the patello-femoral joint; it also forces the quadriceps to strengthen in their least efficient range. The VMO is the major stabiliser of the kneecap against lateral drift.

Figure 9.28 depicts a simple technique, without equipment, used to exercise the VMO strongly. The program is as follows:

1 The patient sits squat by with the trunk supported against the wall, the knee flexed to approximately 60 degrees.
2 This position is held by strong quadriceps contraction until muscle fatigue and tremor begin, approximately 60-90 seconds.
3 Progression is made by increasing time, increasing the angle of the knees to 90 degrees or single leg stance.
4 If pain is experienced around or under the kneecap the exercise must be stopped.

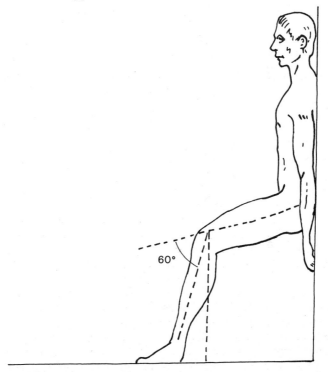

Figure 9.28   The isometric quadriceps position.

Hamstring exercises must be included in any knee rehabilitation. These techniques are described in figure 7.12. When strength and control of the kneecap are achieved, isokinetic procedures for all leg muscles can be introduced to re-develop the strength, power and endurance of the limbs. A graduated return to running is then commenced with careful attention not to overload the offending patello-femoral joint.

The correction of any underlying mechanical or training fault is paramount in the successful management of knee pain. Treatment and rehabilitation will ultimately fail if the underlying problem is not corrected. Running style, surfaces, footwear, training and competition schedules must all be checked by the clinician and corrected where necessary. Pronation and other biomechanical abnormalities may need the care of a sports podiatrist so that the appropriate orthotic control can be dispensed.

Iliotibial Band Friction Syndrome

Iliotibial band friction syndrome (ITBFS) is an overuse injury seen primarily in distance runners and occasionally in other sports such as skiing and cycling.

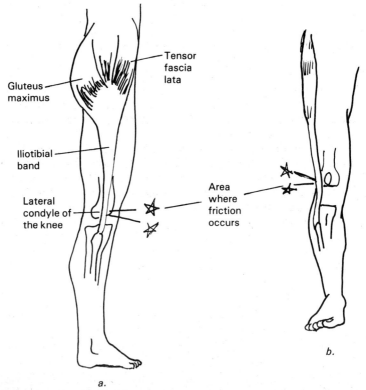

Figure 9.29 The iliotibial band and the site of frictioning on the lateral femoral condyle.

Anatomy

The iliotibial band is a thickening of a band strip of fascial tissue extending from the tensor fascia lata and gluteus maximus muscles at the iliac crest to the outer surface of the lower leg (fig. 9.29). At the knee, the band crosses close to the large outside edge of the femur (lateral condyle). This is the site where friction occurs between the femoral condyle and the iliotibial tract during flexion and extension of the knee whilst running. This frictioning results in inflammation of the iliotibial band, the underlying bursa or the outer surface of the bony condyle (periosteum) (fig 9.29).

Cause of Injury

The major cause of this injury is overuse due to covering long distances and muscle tightness associated with distance running. All distance runners are notorious "non-stretchers" and the limited range of motion of the hip in distance running styles encourages the tightening of the thigh muscles, particularly the iliotibial band. The tight iliotibial band then rubs on the femoral condyle of the knee causing the resultant pain and inflammation and damage.

Training errors, particularly a rapid increase in weekly training or an unusually long run, can precipitate the condition. Runners who run consistently on the same side of the road can develop the pain on the downhill leg. Worn or inappropriate running shoes appear to worsen the problem.

In the authors' experience, many ITBFS patients have presenting anatomical or biomechanical faults. Poor limb alignment and anatomical anomalies such as prominent lateral femoral condyle, tibial torsion, or genu varum are examples. However, the most common presenting problem is the biomechanical imbalance associated with overpronation of the forefoot (see page 242). Internal rotation of the tibia associated with overpronation during running tightens the iliotibial band and also makes the femoral condyle more prominent, causing friction to occur (fig. 9.30).

Signs and Symptoms

Athletes with ITBFS experience pain on the outside of the leg just above the joint line and this can radiate down to the upper part of the lower leg. Classically, the pain appears in runners who cover a constant distance, usually between 3 to 10 kilometres. It disappears when running is stopped, and most sufferers can walk comfortably with no pain; many are able to play other sports such as squash and tennis without discomfort. Running downhill,

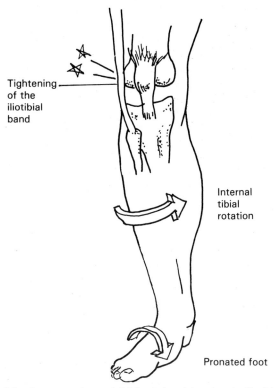

Tightening of the iliotibial band

Internal tibial rotation

Pronated foot

Figure 9.30 Overpronation and tibial rotation tightening the iliotibial band.

walking down stairs or slopes typically worsens the symptoms. The longer the distance the athlete runs the worse the pain becomes, until he or she is forced to stop.

Diagnosis is made by localising the tenderness over the lateral condyle of the femur. This tenderness is more prominent when the knee is flexed to 30 degrees. Normally, there is no history of direct trauma or twisting injury to the knee; therefore there is no significant swelling and all tests for internal derangement of the knee (chapter 7, "Joint injuries") appear negative.

Treatment

The major principle of treatment is to treat the cause, which in most cases is a training error. A reduction of distance, speed, restriction to flat surfaces and a shortening of stride length to within pain-free limits are strictly enforced.

Physiotherapy management is indicated, initially using symptom-relieving modalities such as I.C.E. and various electro-therapeutic agents. The main emphasis of physical therapy should be the assessment and correction of muscle imbalance situations around the thigh. Stretching and rehabilitative exercises for the iliotibial band and other thigh muscles such as the hip flexors, hamstrings and calf muscles should be prescribed. The specific stretches to the iliotibial band are illustrated in figure 9.31.

It is important to note that with knee pain of long standing, the quadriceps muscles can precipitate peripatellar pain. All ITBFS patients should be placed on a quadriceps/hamstring rehabilitation drill to counter quadriceps and hamstring muscle wastage and weakness.

Recovery from this condition can often be protracted, sometimes taking from 2 to 6 months, particularly if there has

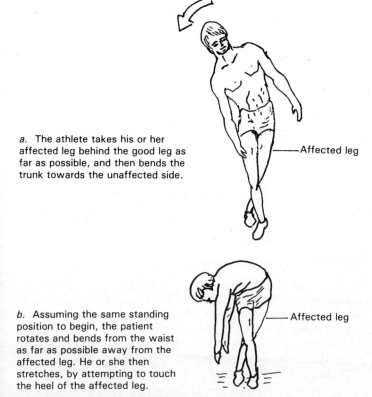

a. The athlete takes his or her affected leg behind the good leg as far as possible, and then bends the trunk towards the unaffected side.

Affected leg

b. Assuming the same standing position to begin, the patient rotates and bends from the waist as far as possible away from the affected leg. He or she then stretches, by attempting to touch the heel of the affected leg.

Affected leg

Figure 9.31   Stretches to the iliotibial band.

c. The patient lies with the affected leg on top, wearing a weight shoe on the foot
(i). The affected leg is held straight and extended over the edge of the table
(ii). The weight plus gravity stretches the iliotibial band and strengthens the damaged area as the weight is lifted and returned to the starting position.

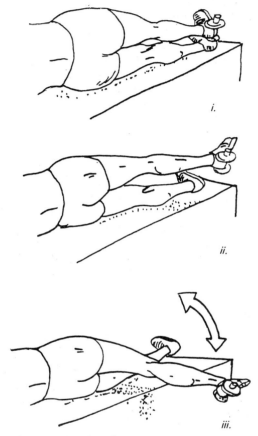

i.

ii.

iii.

Figure 9.31   Stretches (continued).

been periosteal (bony) irritation. Refractory cases may need the assistance of anti-inflammatory medication or cortisone injections to help settle the inflammatory process.

Severe biomechanical imbalances, such as excessive pronation, need the professional attention of a sports podiatrist for appropriate orthotic management.

BACK, HIP AND PELVIC PAIN IN RUNNING ATHLETES

Overuse injuries that occur in this region are very subtle and are usually related to situations such as training errors or biomechanical problems related to muscle imbalance or poor alignment of the lower limb. As well as the standard procedures for examining the low back, hip and pelvis, the clinician must include variables such as pelvic tilt, leg length, femoral neck anteversion alignment and position of the patella, knee configuration (genu valgum, varum, recurvatum), tibial torsion, lower leg/forefoot alignment, arch configuration and shoe wear.

Back Pain in Runners

Back pain is a common affliction of athletes, especially for long distance runners. It is usually an ache of mechanical origin and may develop into a full blown lumbar disc syndrome (see chapter 8 on back pain). Pain arising from the sacroiliac joint may also mimic back pain (see page 290 in this section).

A full examination of the back including a biomechanical examination of the hip, lower limb and feet must be conducted by a sports medicine doctor or sports physiotherapist. This examination may exclude the major causes of back pain discussed in chapter 8 and, therefore, the possibility that back pain could be due to the following subtle causes peculiar to runners must be considered.

The Short Leg Syndrome

Any leg length discrepancy can lead to pelvic tilting and scoliosis as a compensatory mechanism (fig. 9.32). These postural deviations in turn place stress and tension on the lumbar ligaments and other soft tissues supporting the spine, causing their eventual breakdown, inflammation and repair by scar tissue.

The short leg may be functional or of anatomical origin. *Functional short leg* means that the actual leg lengths are the same but one leg appears shorter due to overpronation of one foot relative to the other. The excessive pronation of one foot causes that leg to be "shorter" in standing, allowing lateral pelvic tilt and compensatory scoliosis (fig. 9.33). Correction of this fault can be achieved by the appropriate orthotic device.

Anatomical short leg This means that one leg is actually physically shorter than the opposite leg. The short leg may be due to some birth or hereditary defect or the result of some

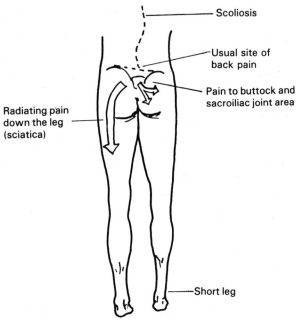

Figure 9.32 Short leg syndrome, with compensatory pelvic tilt and scoliosis.

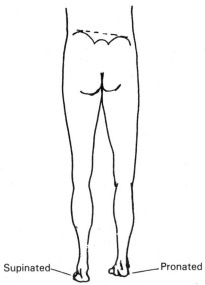

Figure 9.33 Functional short leg.

traumatic insult such as surgery or fracture to the leg bones which leaves the bones shorter. When the leg length discrepancy is greater than 6 mm, a shoe raise may be prescribed to correct the discrepancy.

Bilateral Overpronation

Excessive overpronation of the feet associated with the poor alignment syndrome (figs 9.2 and 9.3) results in forward tilting of the pelvis with excessive lumbar lordosis (inward curve of the spine). The increase in lordosis or "sway back" (fig. 8.11), causes excessive stress to the supporting structures of the spine when running. Correction is achieved by the appropriate orthotic device or shoes and rehabilitative back exercises to correct the lordosis.

Muscle Imbalance

These situations are very common in all runners and athletes (fig. 9.7). In general terms, weakness develops in the abdominals, buttock and back, while excessive tightness occurs in the calf muscles, hamstrings, iliotibial band, hip flexors and back muscles. This lack of strength-flexibility balance can easily predispose to back pain. If the imbalance is bilateral the pelvis will tip forward anteriorly, developing an excessive lordosis. A unilateral imbalance will allow rotation of the pelvis forward and a lateral pelvic tilt towards the affected side. These abnormal postural patterns overstress the supporting structures of the spine and sacroiliac joints causing eventual breakdown and pain.

Piriformis Syndrome

Runners are particularly susceptible to this syndrome. Spasm of the piriformis muscle, which is situated deep within the buttocks, can put pressure on the sciatic nerve giving symptoms down the leg, therefore masquerading as a "pseudo-nerve root irritation". The exact cause of tightness and spasm of the piriformis is unclear. However, it is the authors' experience that it is usually associated with a biomechanical or alignment fault such as overpronation or a muscle imbalance. The condition is treated by specific manual stretches to the piriformis muscle, stretching exercises (fig. 1.3) and correction of the biomechanical fault/muscle imbalance.

Treatment of Back Pain in Runners

The treatment of back pain in runners is to follow the principles of the management of back pain in chapter 8 to provide symptomatic relief and rehabilitation of the damaged soft tissues. However, the successful treatment of runners depends on discovering the precise cause(s) and correcting the problem with the appropriate means.

Hip and Pelvic Overuse Injuries

Few overuse injuries occur to the hip and pelvic region in sport. When they occur they are usually nagging injuries that can plague the athlete for months. Because of this low incidence of the conditions, diagnosis and management are poorly understood.

Bony Injury

True pain of the hip joint(s) is rare. Degenerative changes which develop in the older athlete are the most usual cause. Stress fractures are uncommon in the hip and pelvic region; however, stress fractures at the femoral neck can have devasting consequences. This is because undetected stress fractures can progress to displacement at the fracture site which can damage the fragile blood supply to the ball of the hip joint (femoral head) leading to bony death (avascular necrosis) and subsequent osteoarthritis (fig. 9.34). X-rays may not pick up a stress fracture; therefore, bone-scanning techniques are used for early diagnosis.

Stress fractures may also occur to the pubic bones and stress-related injuries can damage the symphysis pubis. The incidence of injury to the symphysis pubis is usually more related to

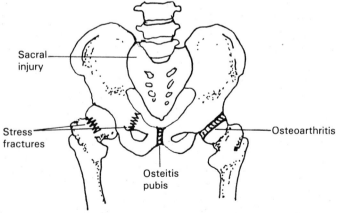

Figure 9.34   Bony overuse injury to hip and pelvis.

traumatic insult and the condition is covered in depth in chapter 7, "Muscular injuries" on traumatic osteitis pubis.

Soft Tissue Injury

The majority of hip-related pain in athletes originates from the surrounding soft tissues. Tissues which are implicated most are the gluteus medius muscle, tensor fascia lata muscle, the iliotibial band and the trochanteric bursa (fig. 9.35). Strains of muscle groups acting on the hip such as the adductors, hamstrings and the quadriceps are common and are covered in depth in chapter 7, "Muscular injuries".

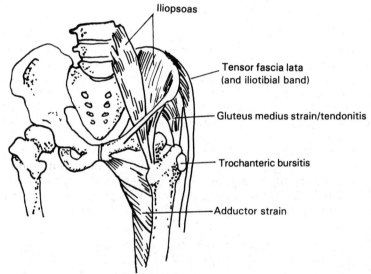

Iliopsoas

Tensor fascia lata (and iliotibial band)

Gluteus medius strain/tendonitis

Trochanteric bursitis

Adductor strain

Figure 9.35   Soft tissue injury to the hip.

The gluteus medius is thought to fatigue quickly if there is an exaggerated sideways tilt or "seesawing" motion of the pelvis. This fatigue to the muscle leads to an inflammatory tendonitis at the tendon of insertion onto the greater trochanter of the hip (fig. 9.35).

Poor running posture with anterior pelvic tilt and sway back (fig. 8.11) will cause hypertrophy and tightness of many muscles acting around the hip, particularly the tensor fascia lata and the iliotibial band. A tight iliotibial band leads to a friction syndrome (similar to iliotibial band friction syndrome of the knee, page 280), onto the trochanteric bursa causing inflammation (bursitis).

Pain is experienced over the lateral aspect of the hip, which is often made worse when running on slopes. The pain begins as a slight discomfort and, if activity is continued, the pain will increase until running and training must be stopped. Tenderness is localised to the greater trochanter of the hip. Tenderness above the greater trochanter and pain on resisted abduction implicate the gluteus medius. Lateral tenderness and no pain on resisted abduction suggest a trochanteric bursitis.

As with all overuse injuries, causative factors in hip pain are a combination of training errors, anatomical factors and environmental factors. All these problems have been discussed in depth throughout this section. It is important for the clinician to realise that overuse hip injuries are often associated with biomechanical faults; therefore, just treating the local problem will not always achieve a favourable result. Short leg syndromes, muscle imbalance situations and lower limb alignment problems, especially when coupled with compensatory pronation, can predispose to hip pain.

Sacroiliac Joint Dysfunction

Vague pain around the hips, low back, thighs, buttocks and upper hamstrings is often associated with dysfunction of the sacroiliac joint (SIJ) (fig. 9.36). This joint was considered to be very stable, but recently more attention is being given to the joint as a source of pain.

Women appear more susceptible to SIJ problems, especially after childbirth. The wider gynecoid pelvis of females can enhance the biomechanical forces generated in sports which act on the hip and pelvis. However, the main reason seems to be the softening of the ligaments of the spine, SIJ and the symphysis pubis to allow childbirth. This situation leaves these structures vulnerable to injury on recommencing sport/vigorous activity after birth. Proper postnatal and restrengthening exercises coupled with a gradual return to activity must be followed to allow the ligamentous structures to return to full strength.

Stress to the SIJ is often associated with muscle imbalance, especially tightness of the adductors, hip flexors and the iliotibial band. Traumatic injury to the SIJ can occur with "impact" sports such as triple jump, long jump, rugby and is sometimes associated with traumatic osteitis pubis (chapter 7, "Muscular injuries").

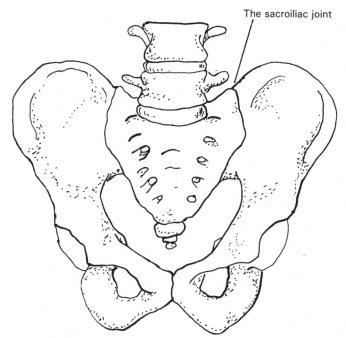

The sacroiliac joint

Figure 9.36 The sacroiliac joint.

Abnormal biomechanics also plays a significant role in the development of SIJ pain. These situations include:
- poor running style and posture which allows excessive up and down tilt of the pelvis and sway back;
- short leg syndromes;
- lateral pelvic tilt and compensatory scoliosis;
- poor limb alignment and compensatory pronation.

Treatment of Hip and Pelvic Pain

In the authors' experience, the recovery time for hip-related problems is often long. The major reason is that in the main they are nagging problems which do not initially prevent activity, and consequently it is some months before correct advice is sought.

Bony injuries and osteitis pubis may need prolonged periods of total rest before even non-weight-bearing exercise, such as swimming and cycling, can be prescribed. As pain subsides, these activities and running in the deeper end of a pool can be begun. Weight-bearing activities can be started only when the athlete is pain-free in ordinary daily activities. Return to sport must be a slow, gradual process.

Treatment of soft-tissue problems consists of local applications of ice and physiotherapy modalities at the site(s) of tenderness. Muscle imbalance situations must be assessed and the appropriate stretching and strengthening rehabilitative exercises prescribed. Tightness of the hamstrings, iliotibial band and hip flexors coupled with weak abdominals and hip extensors (gluteals) is a common finding in hip and pelvic injury. Anatomical and biomechanical factors such as leg length discrepancies, poor limb alignment and compensatory pronation often need the appropriate orthotic appliance to gain a full return to pain-free sport.

Sacroiliac joint dysfunction needs the accurate assessment and management of a trained therapist. Treatment procedures can range from manipulative techniques, SIJ bracing to specialised rehabilitative exercise.

10
INJURIES TO THE SHOULDER AND ELBOW FROM THROWING, SWIMMING AND RACQUET SPORTS

Acute and chronic overuse injuries often affect the elbow and shoulder in sports activities such as throwing a ball, swimming and the serving action in tennis. In this chapter only the more frequent soft tissue injuries that occur to the arm are discussed.

SHOULDER PAIN—THE ROTATOR CUFF IMPINGEMENT SYNDROME

Pain around the shoulder joint in sports usually arises from pathology affecting the components of the rotator cuff complex. Painful arc syndrome, rotator cuff tendonitis, supraspinatus tendonitis and bursitis are some names used to describe pain and dysfunction of the shoulder originating from soft tissue injury. For the purpose of this book, the term "rotator cuff impingement syndrome" will be used to describe this spectrum of pathological entities.

ANATOMY OF THE ROTATOR CUFF

The superficial muscles around the shoulder region are responsible for the gross movements of the shoulder joint (fig. 10.1). The prime movers which extend the shoulder backwards are the latissimus dorsi and the posterior deltoid. Flexing in a forward motion is initiated by the anterior deltoid, while all the fibres of the deltoid acting in conjunction will raise the arm outwards from the body (abduction). The pectoralis major moves the arm horizontally across the body and the trapezius will shrug the shoulder girdle.

Below the superficial muscles are a deeper group collectively called the rotator cuff (fig. 10.2). These muscles are responsible for the intricate movements of the shoulder, such as rotation of the arm during activities such as throwing and swimming. The rotator cuff consists of the subscapularis, supraspinatus,

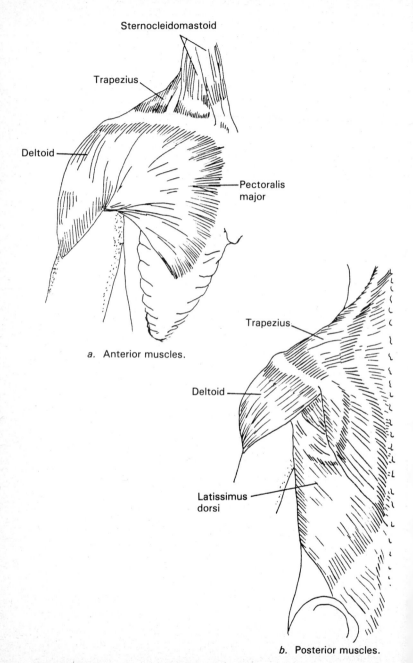

a. Anterior muscles.

b. Posterior muscles.

Figure 10.1 Superficial muscles of the shoulder.

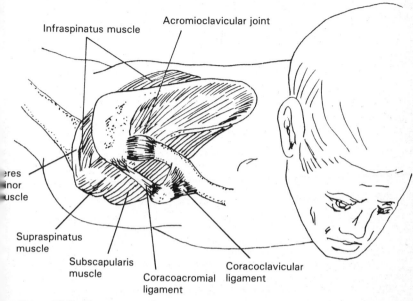

Figure 10.2 The rotator cuff muscles viewed from above.

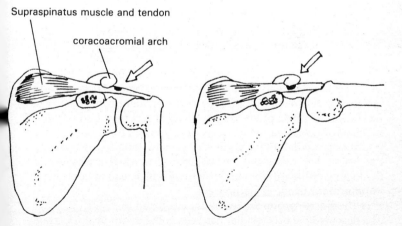

Figure 10.3 Impingement of the supraspinatus muscle under the coracoacromial arch.

infraspinatus and the teres minor muscles. The supraspinatus is the primary muscle involved in rotator cuff impingement syndrome. Other structures which also may be involved include the biceps tendon, the subacromial bursa and the joint capsule.

The supraspinatus and the biceps tendon are highly susceptible to injury because when the arm is elevated, the rotator cuff must function beneath an arch comprised of the bony acromion and the coracoacromial ligament (the coracoacromial arch) (fig. 10.3).

Because of the small clearance between the rotator cuff and the coracoacromial arch, repetitive activity above the horizontal plane can lead to mechanical irritation beneath the arch of the structures of the rotator cuff, such as the supraspinatus tendon, the subacromial bursa and the adjacent biceps tendon (fig. 10.3). Prolonged mechanical irritation will produce pain, inflammation, cellular death and eventual scarring. Table 10.1 illustrates the pathological stages of the condition.

Table 10.1   The pathology of the rotator cuff impingement syndrome.

Stage	Pathology	Prognosis
I	Irritation leading to oedema (swelling) and haemorrhage (bleeding)	Reversible
II	Inflammation of the tendon (tendonitis) and fibrosis (scarring) and thickening	Reversible
III	Degeneration and eventual tearing of the tendon	Often irreversible

Rotator cuff impingement syndrome presents in one of three distinct groups; the highly competitive athlete, the person playing "weekend" or recreational sports and the middle-aged to elderly person.

Competitive and professional athletes usually present with their shoulder problem early (stage 1 pathology) and their symptoms are totally reversible with the correct treatment principles. The recreational athlete often has a prolonged recovery and requires much effort and treatment to return to sport. This is because the injury is ignored until function is extremely impaired. Therefore, the lesion has advanced inflammation, marked scarring and thickening of the rotator cuff structures which lead to continuing impingement (stage II pathology).

In the elderly group the lesion is considered to be the end stage of a degenerative process that has been going on for years. Certain physiological processes involved in ageing appear to make tendons more susceptible to injury. These physiological changes include hormonal changes that occur in women, and the decline of extensibility and strength in muscle and tendon tissues with age. The continuing inflammatory process spreads to other structures, such as the joint capsule, leading to "frozen shoulder", calcification of the supraspinatus tendon and partial or complete tearing of the rotator cuff. The resultant thickening and scarring under the coracoacromial arch may lead to an irreversible condition and surgical procedures may be indicated (stage III pathology).

CAUSE OF INJURY

As with all other overuse syndromes, the primary cause is an error in training. Shoulder pain tends to be recurrent in athletes, the symptoms occurring either in the beginning of the season or near the end. This is because athletes are either trying to upgrade their training too quickly or they are getting tired as the intensity of training and playing increases.

Incorrect technique also plays a dominant role in injury. The correct throwing style can reduce the stress to shoulder and arm. The whipping action of a side arm throw may slightly increase the speed of delivery. However, this technique, particularly when the body opens up too soon in the delivery, will cause excessive stress to the upper limb. Overhead strokes, a miss hit, or trying to put too much spin on the ball in a tennis serve are common injury-producing situations.

In order to understand how the rotator cuff may be injured, it is necessary to understand some basic biomechanics involved in the various sports where rotator cuff lesions are frequent.

Throwing and Racquet Sports

The overhead action involved in these activities can be divided into three phases; the wind-up or cocking phase, the acceleration phase and the follow-through (fig. 10.4).

The acceleration phase is where the explosive force of the action is developed and, consequently, the phase in which most injury occurs. The arm is rapidly moved forward at speed and in addition is whipped from an externally rotated position to an internally rotated position prior to follow-through. This action in a throw or tennis serve/smash places great stress on the rotator cuff muscles and can cause irritation, inflammation and eventual impingement. Overhead action in sport can develop a force exceeding 135 kg which distracts the joint to such an extent that the head of the humerus can leave the socket by up to 3 cm or more. This force can obviously overstretch the capsule, ligaments and muscles maintaining the integrity of the shoulder joint.

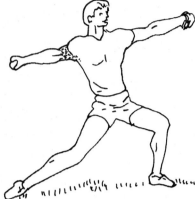

a. Cocking phase.

When cocked preparing to throw, the shoulder is in maximum external rotation.

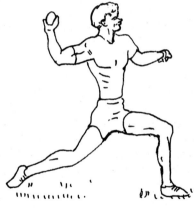

b. Acceleration phase.

This begins with a weight transfer forward; the arm moves rapidly into internal rotation.

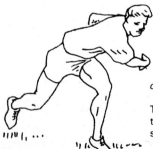

c. Follow through.

The muscles of the arm decelerate the limb, bringing the throw to a smooth halt.

Figure 10.4 The phases of throwing.

Therefore, injury to the structures of the shoulder can occur with excessive, repetitive, explosive overhead activity.

Constant repetitive sports action causes the dominant arm to undergo hypertrophy (an increase in size and strength) in selected muscles, particularly the muscles involved in the acceleration phase such as the anterior deltoid, the pectorals and the subscapularis. Therefore, an imbalance situation can develop where these muscles become stronger and inflexible, whereas the other muscles protecting the shoulder become weak and stretched, leading to eventual injury.

Shoulder dysfunction is very common amongst baseballers, softballers, tennis players and outfield throwers in cricket. Surprisingly, it is not a common injury among cricket bowlers. This is because the side on, straight arm action in bowling places little stress on the shoulder joint, as the force of delivering the ball develops mainly in the trunk muscles and the "run up". The exception to this is the "leg spinner" whose action in turning the ball can cause impingement of the rotator cuff.

Swimming

The shoulder is the most frequently injured anatomical area in swimmers. The competitive swimmer is estimated to use approximately ten thousand strokes, per shoulder, per week and a half a million strokes to each shoulder in a season. It is hardly suprising that overuse injury can result from the long gruelling workouts that swimmers undergo. The incidence of swimmer's shoulder is also known to:
  • increase with age;
  • be more prevalent in freestyle and butterfly;
  • increase with distance; and
  • occur more in the elite athlete.

In modern swimming strokes the upper limb is the prime mover so as training distances and speed increases, the stress to the shoulder also increases. Therefore, improper stroke mechanics play a major role in the development of "swimmer's shoulder". The major fault occurs when the arm is forcefully held in the position of internal rotation during the pull through phase of the stroke. The internally rotated shoulder will cause the biceps tendon and the rotator cuff to impinge on the coracoacromial arch. Freestylers who breathe only over one shoulder can cause excessive stress to the shoulder on the non-breathing side.

Therefore, changing the stroke pattern to enable the swimmer to breathe on alternate sides can correct the problem.

It has been demonstrated that the blood circulation to the biceps tendon and the rotator cuff is compromised during that part of the stroke where impingement occurs between these structures and the coracoacromial arch. Repetitive stress, poor stroke mechanics and the subsequent avascularity (decreased blood supply) will eventually lead to the development of the rotator cuff impingement syndrome.

SIGNS AND SYMPTOMS

Young competitive athletes normally have an insidious onset of soreness after or during activity. The area where the pain is felt is usually below the shoulder joint at the point of insertion of the deltoid (fig. 10.5).

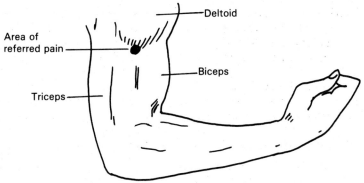

Figure 10.5 The area where tenderness is usually experienced in the rotator cuff impingement syndrome.

Pain increases as the overload activity continues until the pain interferes with function. In the less fit or unskilled athlete there can be one incidence of trauma (such as, a miss hit of an overhead smash in tennis) which is painful for some time after the incident. The pain usually subsides in a day or two, only to return at the next attempt at sport. Table 10.2 illustrates the various stages in the development of symptoms.

The older patient will complain of an aching pain, particularly at rest. Acute pain can occur during the performance of simple tasks carried out in the horizontal plane or overload. Because of protective postures and with the progressing pathology, these

Table 10.2   The stages in the development of symptoms in the rotator cuff impingement syndrome.

Stage	Symptoms
I	Pain develops after activity.
II	Pain begins to occur with activity, but the athlete can continue with no decrease in performance.
III	The athlete continues to play, but pain significantly decreases performance.
IV	The athlete cannot compete and experiences continued pain, even at rest.

patients present with increasing stiffening of the shoulder and greatly diminished function. Simple tasks such as dressing become painful and difficult to accomplish.

The classic clinical sign in advanced rotator cuff impingement is the movement of the arm outwards into abduction. This action will produce a "painful arc" when the swollen scarred rotator cuff impinges against the bone of the coracoacromial arch. The movement is pain-free in the initial stages, becoming painful during impingement, and then pain-free again as the rotator cuff moves under the arch (fig. 10.6).

The diagnosis of the various rotator cuff injuries requires the training and skill of an experienced clinician. Many tests and examination procedures must be carried out to identify the particular structure damaged so that the appropriate rehabilitation program can be prescribed. Other tests must also be given to eliminate shoulder pain originating from other sources, such as cervical and thoracic spine pathology, stress fracture, recurrent dislocation, and so on.

TREATMENT

The treatment of shoulder pain is based on three major principles consistently discussed throughout this book.

1 Symptomatic Relief

The primary aim is to decrease the inflammatory response and hence decrease the pain and discomfort. As always I.C.E. is the modality of choice in the acute phase. Activity of the shoulder must be limited to pain-free movements. If pain-producing activity is continued, there will be increased inflammation, increased impingement and therefore, more damage and scarring which may

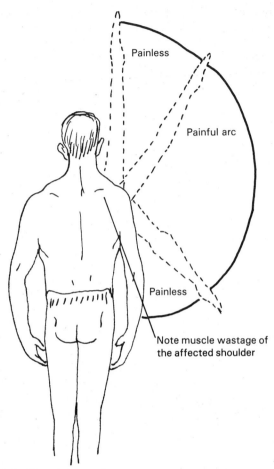

Figure 10.6   The painful arc sign.

inhibit complete recovery. If the condition has been allowed to progress, intensive physiotherapy will be needed. Refractory cases may need anti-inflammatory medication prescribed either orally or by injection.

2 Rehabilitation

Isometric exercises must be instigated immediately to maintain muscle strength when active movement of the shoulder causes acute pain (fig. 6.3). As inflammation is brought under control and there is no pain at rest, pain-free range of motion exercises can be commenced. With elderly patients and the severely injured athlete, gravity-free or assisted/active movements using devices such as pulley systems may be indicated (fig. 6.4).

When the range of motion improves and the pain subsides, isotonic exercises can be prescribed. The program must be tailored to each injury and must avoid the repetitive tasks that caused the initial damage. These isotonic exercises are done with free weights, such as dumbbells, so that all combinations of shoulder movements can be exercised. Suitable exercises are described in figure 6.5. An important exercise that must be included is the "upsidedown beer can" exercise (fig. 10.7) which isolates the supraspinatus muscle.

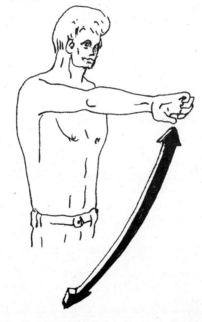

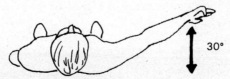

Figure 10.7 The supraspinatus exercise.

All isotonic exercises must begin with light weights and few repetitions, progressing as pain and function allows. Isokinetic exercises on special apparatus, such as the Cybex, are the final stage to develop the power and endurance parameters for sport.

Once strength and movement are gained through the rehabilitation program, a return to the functional activities of sport is commenced. A slow, gradual return to full sport participation is essential. If the return to sport is too quick, the healing structures can be easily overloaded and re-injured.

The program described is usually all that is required to return the young competitive athlete to sport. The recreational athlete and the older patient will often need intensive physiotherapy to treat the scarring and loss of range of motion that occurs in the chronic injury. As well as the electrotherapy modalities, specialised stretches and shoulder joint mobilisations are required to restore function to the shoulder joint.

3 Correction of the Fault

Failure to correct the mechanical cause of the injury is usually the reason for the failure of a treatment program. In problem cases it is extremely important to observe the athlete's action to determine the problem area. Videotaping the athlete and analysing the film can be a very useful way to identify the problem motion.

Training programs must be monitored closely, as a mistake in training load can easily cause injury. Fatigue plays a significant role in the development of overuse syndromes. Mistakes include upgrading a training schedule too quickly, not allowing sufficient rest and returning to training at too high a level after a layoff.

THE PREVENTION OF SHOULDER OVERUSE INJURIES

1 Flexibility

A year-round flexibility program for the shoulder and upper body must be maintained. Slow static stretching as described in chapter 1 (fig. 1.1) should be conducted. It is important in the throwing shoulder to increase the range of motion of the external rotators and extensors.

2 Strength, Power and Endurance

Overuse injuries around the shoulder are often considered to be due to muscle imbalance caused by the hypertrophy of the muscles involved as prime movers of the sports action. To prevent this imbalance situation it is important for the athlete to undergo a regular weight-training program, especially pre-season, to develop and maintain the strength, power and endurance of all muscles acting on the shoulder and upper body. If specific problems are apparent the athlete should seek a sports physiotherapist to conduct muscle-testing procedures to identify the muscle imbalance and prescribe the necessary retraining exercises.

3 Warm-up and Care of the Shoulder

The principles of a "warm-up" discussed in chapter 1 should be followed. Specific factors to undertake with the shoulder are:
- gentle, slow, static stretching of the upper limb and trunk before activity;
- performing the throwing/racquet action gently without the ball;
- gradually introducing the ball and slowly increasing the velocity and power of the action until full power is achieved;
- after competition, performing gentle stretches and exercises in a warm-down;
- if any pain or soreness is apparent after competition applying I.C.E. and seeking the appropriate medical attention.

4 Technique

As discussed previously, improper technique or stroke play is a primary cause of injury. This is particularly evident with weekend and recreational athletes. Good coaching imparts the proper techniques of sport and this is extremely important in preventing the overuse syndromes.

THE ELBOW "OVERUSE" SYNDROMES

THROWER'S ELBOW (medial collateral ligament sprain)

Elbow injury in throwing sports usually develops from a valgus (outward) force to the joint. This causes an opening stress onto the medial (inside) structures of the elbow and compressive forces to the lateral side of the joint (fig. 10.8).

Many conditions can occur in the elbow as a result of excessive

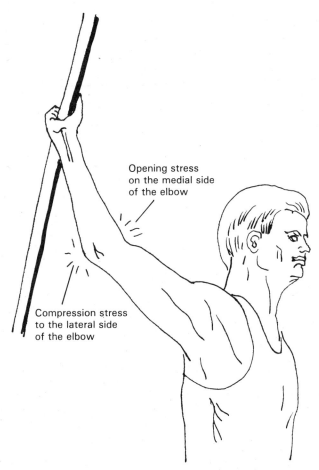

Figure 10.8   Valgus overload on the elbow of a thrower.

throwing, especially coupled with poor technique. Table 10.3 provides a summary of the various pathologies that may develop.

However, the predominant lesion in thrower's elbow is a sprain of the medial collateral ligament. This ligament straps the humerus to the ulna and helps to stabilise the joint against valgus forces (fig. 10.9).

Cause of Injury

Over-stress to the medial collateral ligament is primarily caused

Table 10.3 Elbow pathologies from throwing.

Medial side	Lateral side
Musculotendinous strain of the wrist flexor origin (see ''golfer's elbow'').	Musculotendinous strain of the wrist extensor origin (see ''tennis elbow'').
Medial epicondylar fracture	Avulsion fracture
Ulnar nerve intrapment	Loose bodies
Soft tissue calcification	
Medial collateral ligament sprain	

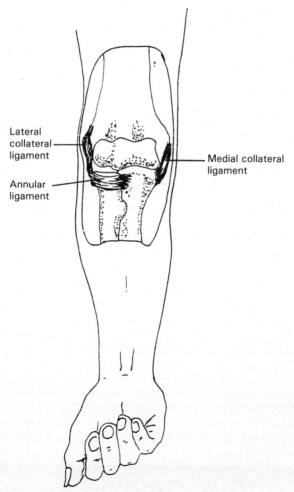

Figure 10.9 The ligaments of the right elbow, viewed from the front.

by poor technique, particularly the "round arm throw". In this type of delivery, the elbow is bent and leads the shoulder in the acceleration phase of throwing. The forces involved in this throw open up the inside of the elbow, damaging the medial collateral ligament of the joint (fig. 10.8). Repetitive poor throws will cause inflammation, ligament tissue death and repair by scar tissue. Sports where this injury is prevalent include baseball, softball and the javelin throw.

Signs and Symptoms

Initially, pain is felt on the inside of the elbow on throwing and ceases after activity. If throwing is continued, the pain will increase until it is experienced with activity or even at rest. The untreated elbow will develop decreases in elbow motion, particularly when the patient is attempting to straighten the joint fully. Full elbow extension is quite painful. Slight effusion (swelling) is often observed over the medial collateral ligament. Valgus stressing of the joint will reproduce the pain.

Treatment

Symptomatic relief is achieved through the application of the I.C.E. regime and the modification of throwing to within pain-free limits. If symptoms persist, the injury should be vigorously treated with physiotherapy modalities of palliative electrotherapy, mobilising and stretching techniques.

Once symptoms have subsided, rehabilitative exercises to regain the strength, power and endurance of the elbow joint should be instigated. General elbow rehabilitative exercises are discussed in the following section on "Tennis elbow".

A general program of strengthening and stretching exercises to the wrist, shoulder and upper trunk should be maintained throughout injury rehabilitation.

Sprains of the medial collateral ligament are caused by repetitive poor technique; unless the technique of throwing is corrected, treatment will fail. This is especially true with the javelin throw. Throwing the javelin exerts considerable stress on the elbow because of the weight of the javelin and the forces produced by the running delivery. Unless the style of delivery is totally correct, injury will invariably result. The forearm must be kept vertical during the acceleration phase of throwing and the elbow should not be allowed to bend into the valgus position.

TENNIS ELBOW (epicondylitis)

"Tennis elbow" is a condition that is not only common amongst athletes, but also occurs in many vocations. The term itself is misleading as it suggests that only tennis players are susceptible to the malady. The elbow is notoriously susceptible to injury from repetitive tasks. Tennis elbow can be brought about by any activity involving repeated forceful grips, especially combined with rotation of the forearm, such as using a screwdriver or painting. These activities demand the same action of the forearm muscles as does the tennis stroke. Therefore, any occupation, hobby, home task or sport involving the repetition of such movements can cause tennis elbow.

The term "tennis elbow", like the term "shin splints", is misleading in that it does not depict a particular ailment. There are many conditions that can cause pain in the vicinity of the elbow, such as nerve entrapment, various bony pathologies and bursitis. In this text, the term "tennis elbow" will be used to describe pain arising from the common wrist and finger extensor muscular origin on the outside of the elbow at the lateral epicondyle (fig. 10.10) and pain on the inside of the elbow arising from the common wrist and finger flexor muscular origin at the medial epicondyle (fig. 10.11).

What is "Tennis Elbow"?

The medical term usually applied to "tennis elbow" is epicondylitis. It refers to a painful inflammation of the tendons of origin in the forearm muscles; the wrist and finger extensors on the lateral side (lateral epicondylitis) and the wrist and finger flexors on the medial side (medial epicondylitis). Repetitive overload causes microtears to these tendons. This damage will lead to inflammation (tendonitis).

Causes of Injury

The overriding factor in the development of tennis elbow is overuse, coupled with poor technique, which produces a force overload to the forearm muscles. If body mechanics, technique and equipment are not right, excessive forces can be placed on the body's tissues. Other factors which play a role in tennis elbow include: the frequency of play, age and sex, and poor levels of conditioning and fitness.

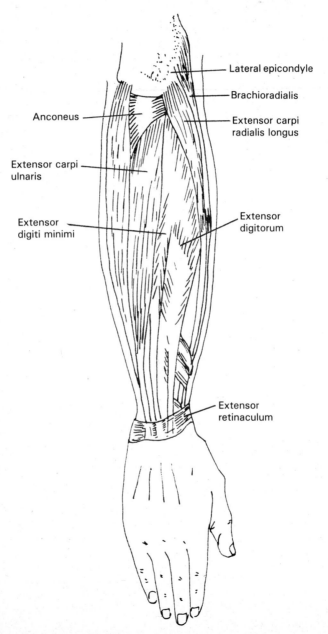

Figure 10.10 The extensor muscles of the forearm, originating at the lateral epicondyle.

Labels (clockwise):
- Lateral epicondyle
- Brachioradialis
- Extensor carpi radialis longus
- Extensor digitorum
- Extensor retinaculum
- Extensor digiti minimi
- Extensor carpi ulnaris
- Anconeus

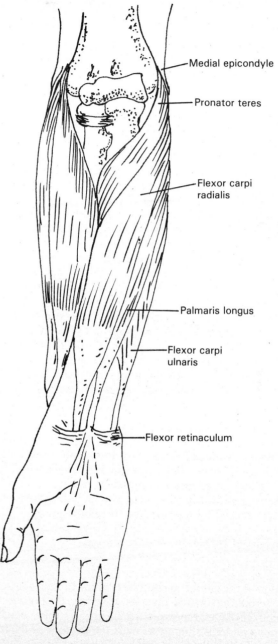

Figure 10.11 The flexor muscles of the forearm, originating at the medial epicondyle.

Frequency of Play

The most likely candidate to suffer from tennis elbow is the middle-aged player of average ability who plays two or three times a week. The harmful effects of poor technique and overuse are cumulative, so that regular playing can cause eventual injury. On the other hand, professional players suffer little from tennis elbow because of their superior fitness and excellent stroke play.

Age and Sex

Tennis elbow rarely occurs before 20 years of age. Members of the 30-to-50 year age group are the most susceptible. In these middle years certain physiological changes occur as part of the ageing process. The body's tissues, especially the tendons, lose their flexibility and muscular strength and endurance begin to decline. Yet the enthusiasm of youth has not been tempered by maturity. As a result, middle-aged players overuse their arms and stress tissues which have begun to lose their resilience.

Women are far more susceptible to the development of tennis elbow than men. Again the ageing process is implicated, particularly the hormonal changes that affect women in mid-life. Deficiencies in the hormone oestrogen may have some relation to degenerative changes that occur in the musculotendinous structures of the body. Therefore, the decrease in muscle elasticity through ageing and hormonal changes is probably responsible for the large numbers of middle-aged female tennis players who suffer from tennis elbow.

Fitness and Conditioning

It is necessary to have a fit, well trained body to withstand the stresses of tennis when played at regular intervals. Weak forearm muscles, a lack of endurance, muscular imbalance or a lack of flexibility will obviously be associated with a decreased resistance to damage caused by overload of the elbow joint.

Mechanisms of Injury

Lateral Side

The region of the lateral epicondyle is prone to injury in activities which overuse the forearm muscles. In tennis, the poor technique of the average player, especially the backhand stroke coupled with poor timing and miss hits, overloads the tendons of the forearm extensors where they originate on the lateral epicondyle.

A poor backhand is delivered with the weight on the back foot and a leading elbow which, with the wrist, is bent and moving at the time of contact with the ball. In this situation the force of the ball is met with a bent elbow held in front of the body and the backhand shot is played with a sudden straightening of the elbow coupled with a snap extension of the wrist. Therefore, instead of the power being derived from the shoulder and trunk, it comes from the forearm extensor muscles; their strength is not adequate to overcome the forces involved in the stroke, so injury must eventuate (fig. 10.12).

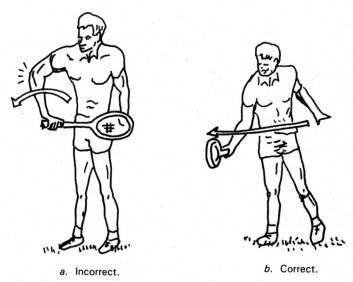

a. Incorrect.   b. Correct.

Figure 10.12   The backhand tennis stroke.

The service action can also be a contributing factor in the development of lateral epicondylitis. This is particularly evident in men who develop large forearm muscles but lack flexibility in the wrist. Any muscle group that develops in size and strength loses flexibility unless specific measures are undertaken to gain and maintain flexibility. In a serve when extra power is required, a wrist snap is executed at the time of impact with the ball. Due to the lack of flexibility of the forearm muscles, this wrist snap easily creates a stretch injury to the point of origin of the muscles on the outside of the elbow.

Medial Side

Medial epicondylitis is more prevalent among the "expert" players, particularly those attempting to impact "top spin" to the ball in a forehand shot. Many players attempt top spin by rolling the racquet head over the ball on impact. The ball is on the racquet head for about 0.004 of a second so there is no way that the racquet can roll over the ball. All that this type of stroke does is stress the medial forearm muscles excessively producing eventual injury. In analysing the game of top tournament players it becomes obvious that the arm motion is not a "roll over", but a natural follow-through starting the stroke low and ending it high, producing the top spin.

The serve can also be implicated in medial epicondylitis. Again men are predominantly affected. The injury is stress related as men tend to attempt to serve harder than women, overloading the medial muscles. Stress to the inside of the elbow can also be magnified if the player attempts to achieve a twist service action.

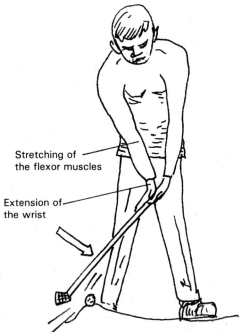

Stretching of the flexor muscles

Extension of the wrist

Figure 10.13 "Golfer's elbow". The club head is blocked by a divot and the wrist is extended forcibly, overstretching the flexor muscles.

GOLFER'S ELBOW (medial epicondylitis)

Medial epicondylitis is often called "golfer's elbow". Figure 10.13 illustrates the mechanism of injury that is common in golf.

Signs and Symptoms

Symptoms usually develop insidiously and become progressively worse until play must cease. Occasionally, injury can occur from a single poorly executed shot, particularly a miss hit. The symptoms usually start with slight discomfort during the performance of a stroke. As the condition worsens, the pain becomes quite severe on completion of a game. The last stage is where a constant ache is felt, even at rest. This pain flares up in any activity involving the forearm muscles.

Tenderness is localised to a specific area on the condyle. Figure 10.14 depicts the point of tenderness that is elicited by palpation of the lateral epicondyle. A similar point can be elicited on the medial epicondyle if the medial forearm muscles are damaged.

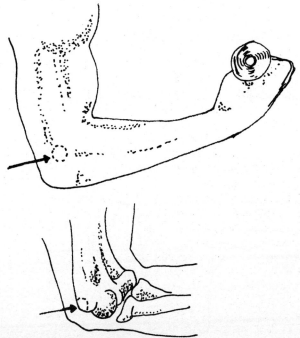

Figure 10.14   The point of tenderness on the lateral condyle of the elbow.

Weakness of the forearm muscles is a sign constantly present with advanced cases. This muscle weakness can be demonstrated by clinical muscle-testing procedures. A very good guide is testing grip strength with a hand dynamometer (fig. 6.13) and comparing the reading to the unaffected side. This procedure can be a handy guide to the effectiveness of the rehabilitation process. The weakness of the forearm muscles is primarily due to pain which limits the use of the muscles, causing them to lose tone, strength and endurance. This situation is termed "disuse atrophy". Many patients complain that this weakness is so advanced that even simple activities, such as picking up a cup of coffee, are impossible.

Chronic cases also display a marked decrease in the flexibility of the wrist and elbow joints (fig. 10.15). This lack of flexibility is an indication of previous injuries which have healed poorly, resulting in a chronically painful scar with its inherent qualities of tightness and weakness. Tennis elbows in this state are very difficult to manage and to achieve any result requires months of hard work and patience under expert guidance.

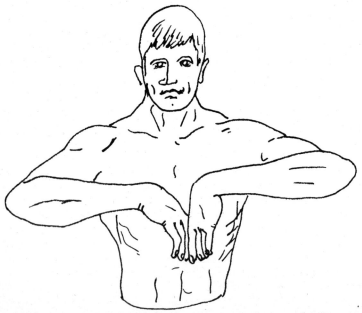

Figure 10.15   Limitation of forearm flexibility, due to shortening and scarring.

Treatment

Tennis elbow is a soft tissue injury of the musculotendinous origin of the forearm muscles; therefore the key to successful treatment is to allow the healing scar to achieve a mature form with all the components of strength, power, endurance and flexibility. In chronic tendonitis the healing process has never been completed and the scar formation is constantly disrupted by the overload forces. The more chronic the condition is, the less chance there is for a favourable prognosis.

The basic treatment approach to tennis elbow is to follow five logical steps:
1 Relieve pain and inflammation.
2 Promote healing of the injury.
3 Regain the strength, power, endurance and flexibility of both arm and forearm.
4 Reduce the overload forces to the elbow which cause the injury to occur.
5 Allow a graduated return to sport.

If each of these steps is not followed to its conclusion, the treatment of tennis elbow will fail.

1   Relief of Inflammation and Pain

Acute phase   The familiar approaches to reducing pain and inflammation discussed continually through this book apply to tennis elbow. Ice applications and modified rest are the treatments of choice. Elevation and compression are usually not necessary as the amount of swelling is insignificant. Acupuncture and various physiotherapy modalities may help to reduce the acute pain.

Tennis elbow should never be totally immobilised, as this leads to muscle atrophy and weakness. Modified rest implies the elimination of any activity that causes pain; for example, with most lateral tennis elbows, the backhand shot causes pain. Therefore, the patient may still play social tennis, avoiding the backhand or any other shot that evokes pain until healing is achieved. It is important to realise that total rest will not resolve tennis elbow, because the healing achieved will be weak and inflexible. It is common to see patients who have rested their elbows for months or even a year, only to have the pain return as soon as they restart tennis.

Chronic phase   Chronic pain and disability need a more sophisticated approach. Anti-inflammatory medication is often needed, prescribed by the doctor. The medication will reduce the inflammation and make the injury feel better, but will not in any way promote healing. Cortisone injections may also be contemplated. The authors believe that these injections are an extreme measure and should be rarely used in the initial treatment. Occasionally, cortisone injections are indicated in the later stages of the treatment program when the pain cycle has not responded totally to conservative measures. At this stage the injury has almost healed, with strength and flexibility returning, but with some residual, resistant pain. Cortisone may be successful in eliminating this residual pain, allowing the rehabilitation process to be completed.

Intensive physiotherapy is also indicated in this chronic phase. Electrotherapeutic modalities, mobilising techniques and acupuncture can help provide symptomatic relief.

2   Promotion of Healing

Healing of any soft tissue injury is the process of allowing scar tissue to grow and mature into a strong, flexible entity. As discussed throughout this book, healing is related to blood flow to the healing tissues. Unfortunately, blood flow to tendons is poor and therefore, healing rates with tendon injuries, such as tennis elbow, are extremely slow. The age, sex and healing capacity of the individual can also have a bearing on healing. The middle-aged to older female group, from experience, are the slowest to heal. In acute cases that are expertly dealt with, after the appearance of pain it usually takes from four to eight weeks to achieve a successful result. In the chronic tennis elbow, many months of patient, diligent work is required. The criteria for successful healing include absence of pain, return to full flexibility and a complete return to strength, power and endurance of the arm muscles.

Physiotherapy modalities such as ultrasound, diathermy and galvanic stimulation coupled with the rehabilitative exercise program are the best methods of promoting healing. Exercise alone will increase blood flow approximately nine times that achieved by expensive machinery. Although premature exercise may be harmful, it is the authors' belief that controlled exercise is the key to stimulate the healing process.

3   Regaining Strength, Power, Endurance and Flexibility

The intensity and timing of the exercise parameters given are critical to the ultimate success of the treatment of tennis elbow. Exercise is difficult to monitor, as pain is the only indication of overload. Therefore, experience and the appropriate education should ensure the safe prescription of therapeutic exercise. Pain and inflammation must be controlled before strong resistance training can begin. A simple indicator is that when a patient can tolerate a moderate handshake, resistance training can begin. A simple method of monitoring strength progress is grip testing using the hand dynamometer (fig. 6.13).

The exercise program should consist of an isotonic regime for the forearm flexors, extensors and rotators. Progressive weight increments are used until three to five kilograms is achieved. Figure 10.16 depicts the various exercises.

Isokinetic exercises to gain maximum power and endurance are added to the isotonic strength program. Specialised devices are necessary to develop these parameters. With the highly competitive or the professional player, emphasis should be placed on high speed training and skill development as opposed to a high weight, low repetition schedule. This is necessary to develop the fast, powerful motor responses required for competition.

In addition to the specific forearm exercises, begin a complete upper body and trunk program to maintain and improve the parameters of fitness. Cardiovascular training must be given to the skilled athlete to maintain his or her competitive edge.

Rehabilitative exercises should be preceded by a comprehensive flexibility routine for the trunk, shoulder, elbow and wrist (refer to the section on flexibility, fig. 1.1. and fig. 1.2). Where specific muscle tightness and inflexibility are evident, specialised physiotherapeutic stretching and mobilising techniques are indicated to restore full function. The total training program must be carried out daily and flexibility and strength gains should be measured and monitored periodically.

The clinical signs of healing are: the complete return to full strength, power, endurance, and a full range of motion with the absence of pain. The dominant arm should be five to ten per cent stronger than the non-playing arm.

4   Reduction of the Overload Forces which Cause Tennis Elbow

Once healing has been achieved, it is paramount to eliminate the overload forces that initially caused the injury to prevent a reoccurrence of the pain. Overload forces can be reduced by three techniques: modifying the player's equipment, forearm bracing

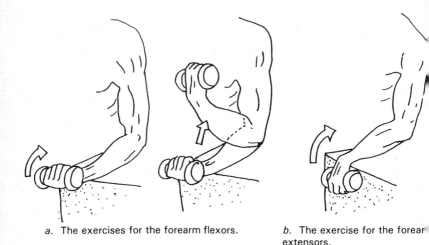

a. The exercises for the forearm flexors.

b. The exercise for the forear extensors.

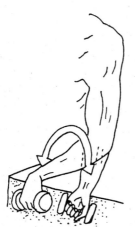
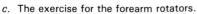

c. The exercise for the forearm rotators.

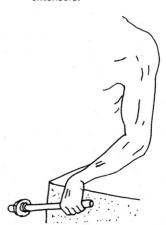

d. Functional exercise to retrain the weaker movements.

Figure 10.16   Strengthening exercises for "tennis elbow".

and modifying the player's technique. These factors, coupled with fitness parameters, are the major concepts in preventing tennis elbow in players without problems.

Equipment modification   Most experts advise a mid-size graphite racquet. Graphite absorbs shock better than other materials used in racquet manufacture. The mid-size racquets have a larger "sweet zone" (the area on the strings where little impact shock is generated) than the standard racquet, therefore reducing the chance of miss hits. The weight of the racquet is also an important consideration. Heavy cheap racquets overload the forearm muscles, leading to muscle fatigue and injury. Light racquets reduce forearm stress and also enable the player to get in position early so that hitting the ball late or miss hitting doesn't occur. The average weight of the lighter racquet best suited to recreational players is 350 g approximately.

Incorrect string tension can play a role in the development of tennis elbow. It is a mistake to string the racquet too tightly. Tight stringing allows greater impact shock forces to be transmitted to the forearm. The recommended tension range in normal racquets appears to be between 25 and 27 kg. Oversized racquets require more initial tension to allow for the increase in area. Gut is thought to be more resilient and protective as a racquet string. However, gut has a limited life and is expensive to replace. Nylon stringing

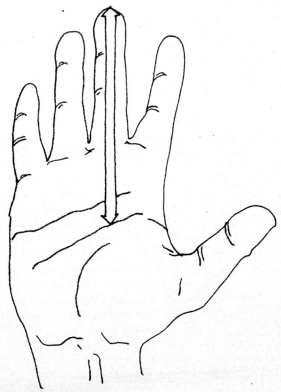

Figure 10.17   Determining the grip size.

is more economical and 16 gauge is recommended for the recreational player.

Theoretically, the larger the grip size, the better the control. The largest handle that a player's hand can comfortably accommodate should be the grip of choice. Smaller grip sizes encourage the "death grip" where the fingers are wrapped tightly around the handle. This type of grip increases the strain on the forearm muscles, especially with a miss hit. Grip size can be determined by measuring from the tip of the ring finger to a point on the lateral crease on the palm between the ring and middle finger (fig. 10.17).

Care must be taken in choosing a new racquet. The choice of an inappropriate grip size, weight or construction of the racquet can easily predispose to tennis elbow. Advice should be sought from qualified tennis professionals.

Forearm bracing   Applying a tennis elbow brace to the forearm is thought to diminish the stressful forces on the elbow. This brace should be of a non-elastic construction with a velcro strap hookup so that tension can be easily adjusted. The brace should be applied so that it is totally comfortable when the muscles are at rest. Tension should only be experienced when the muscles contract (fig. 10.18).

In theory, forearm bracing constrains full muscle expansion thereby diminishing the force generated by the forearm muscles. This small reduction in the muscle force developed, when magnified by hundreds of repetitions, becomes significant in reducing overload forces to the elbow.

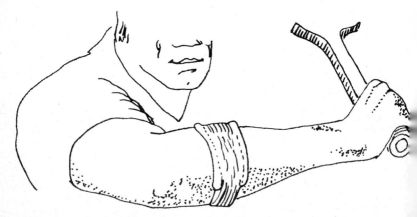

Figure 10.18   Brace for "tennis elbow".

The brace also has a role in rehabilitation. Patients often find that they can perform their exercise routines with more comfort when wearing the brace. The use of the brace is encouraged until the completion of the rehabilitation process; however, most patients continue to use the brace as a preventative measure.

Stroke modification   The onset of tennis elbow is, in most cases, precipitated by poor stroke mechanics overloading the forearm muscles and the elbow. Therefore, modifying the faulty stroke is the most important element in the long-term prevention of reinjury.

The basic principle underlying stroke modification is the transfer of overload forces from the forearm and elbow to the stronger muscles of the shoulder, trunk and upper body. In our experience the most troublesome stroke is the backhand, causing lateral epicondylitis. This situation is particularly evident in the middle-aged to older groups, especially women. Current thought seems to suggest that the two-handed backhand is effective in treating and preventing tennis elbow. Skilled players have problems with the serve or the forehand and usually present with medial epicondylitis. These athletes only need slight adjustments to their stroke mechanics to eradicate the problem.

Modifying a player's technique can be a relatively costly and time-consuming process. It involves the expertise of a qualified tennis coach and, with top level players, the use of video and computer equipment may be necessary to correct the subtlety of a stroke. However, the authors stress the point that if a long term solution to tennis elbow is desired the correction of the problem stroke is paramount.

5 Graduated Return to Sport

All too often players return to hard tennis when the symptoms have abated, only to have their pain and disability return quickly. As stressed throughout this book, a maturing scar should only be exposed to *progressive* overloading. The magic figure is approximately a 10 per cent increase in load per week. Return to full competitive fitness should require a few weeks of careful practice, taking care not to overload and reinjure the elbow. This retraining period can be used profitably in modifying the problem stroke mechanics.

11
MUSCULOSKELETAL PROBLEMS OF CHILDREN IN SPORT

The western world has rediscovered the value of physical exercise; consequently children are participating in organised sports as opposed to play activities at earlier ages and in increasing numbers. Children as young as six have completed marathons; swimmers churn up thousands of metres a day in the pool, young tennis players are set hours of court drill hitting ground strokes and volleys, and so on. Today, young children are becoming so intensely involved in highly organised sports programs that they often require year-long practice and competition. There is also a tendency for children to specialise in one sport at an early age. The pressure from schools, clubs, coaches, parents and peers to train long hours to compete and win can place undue physical and psychological stress on the athlete's growing body.

In view of this increased physical and psychological loading there is a growing concern in the sports medicine fraternity that the limits of the growing skeleton can be exceeded during excessive training and competition. Elite competition and the necessary extreme training at early ages increase the risk of overuse injury. This type of injury is a chronic inflammatory condition caused by repeated microtrauma from repetitive activity. A full discussion of overuse injury and its causes is given in the introduction to part IV. Highly competitive contact sports in the young can expose children to severe traumatic injuries, which may leave permanent impairment, such as joint instability.

Few scientific studies have researched the long term effects of injury to the growing musculoskeletal system, because highly competitive involvement in sport is a relatively recent phenomenon. The fact that a few genetically exceptional individuals are capable of withstanding the extreme training loads of "elite" competition, such as at the Olympic and Commonwealth Games, does not mean that the bulk of our young athletes will not suffer temporary or permanent injury when exposed to long term training loads.

THE EFFECTS OF EXERCISE ON CHILDREN

Recent studies on the effects of exercise on growing bones indicate that exercise regimes within "tolerable limits" stimulate and enhance normal growth. In healthy children the positive growth stimulating effects and general well being associated with physical activity far outweighs the potential risks in a well controlled program. However, the borderline between training loads that are beneficial and training loads that are too stressful (inducing injury) is difficult to define. This is because of the large variance in size, shape, physical condition and maturation levels in children of similar age groups. Unfortunately, when training and competition become too excessive for the young athlete the beneficial effects on the musculoskeletal system are lost and overuse injury will occur which may in turn disrupt normal growth.

Long term physical loading stimulates bony and muscular hypertrophy (increase in size and strength). This situation under normal circumstances is beneficial, as the individual increases in size, strength and physical development. Muscles that undergo hypertrophy increase the cross-sectional area and decrease their length. Therefore, muscle development associated with heavy training and coupled with growth can cause excessive tightness in muscles, especially when flexibility training is inadequate or non-existent. This situation will lead to overuse injuries to the muscles themselves, tendon tissue, joint structures and the growth plates. Problems may also arise in unilateral sports such as tennis and throwing games where overdevelopment may occur on the dominant side which may lead to postural anomalies such as a compensatory scoliosis (see chapter 8).

There is recent scientific evidence that long term high intensity physical loading, such as long distance running, may in fact slow skeletal growth by damaging the growth plates. A bone may sacrifice its growth plate if overloaded by strong continuous forces. Therefore, premature closure of the growth plates may occur causing retardation of growth. The American Academy of Paediatrics has suggested that under no circumstances should a marathon be attempted by immature inidividuals. Once pubertal development is complete the guidelines used for adult distance runners are then appropriate.

A question that is constantly posed by parents to the authors is: "Are weights harmful to children?" Weightlifting is a competitive sport divided into two streams, the Olympic lifts (clean and jerk and the snatch) and the power lifts (dead lift, bench press, squat). The authors believe that pre-adolescent children should not be exposed to the maximum lifts these sports require because of the risks of growth plate damage. If children are interested in these sports they should be encouraged to lift submaximal loads, concentrating on learning the correct techniques and safety in lifting. Once growth is complete, the heavy training required for competition can be commenced.

Training with weights, on the other hand, as opposed to "true" weightlifting, is a method of conditioning using submaximal loads. Programs are designed to enhance performance and aid injury prevention by increasing strength, power and endurance. However, there is probably little to gain for young children until the sex hormones (testosterone and other androgens) are released at puberty. Young children should concentrate on learning the correct lifting skills, safety in using equipment, using light weights to enhance endurance and power and incorporating a well designed flexibility program to supplement the weights. Heavy training, such as low repetition, high load strength sets, should be avoided until growth is complete.

High levels of physical activity also may have an effect on the onset of puberty and reproductive function. Intense exercise can affect certain hormonal responses and, combined with low body fat in a trained individual, cause delayed breast development and menstruation. This prolonged pre-pubescence may also affect skeletal growth, in the relatively long legs seen in elite female track and field athletes and dancers, since, at pre-pubescence, the legs grow faster than the trunk.

Psychological "burnout" is a problem confronting coaches of high level competitive child athletes. Burnout is a condition produced by working too hard and too long in a highly demanding situation. The athlete develops a progressive loss of interest and lacks the desire to train and win. Many children retire from competitive sport long before they reach their physical prime. Some athletes, particularly swimmers, gymnasts and tennis players, have trained constantly for nearly a decade by the time they reach 17.

Obviously, not every young athlete who works long and hard under pressure experiences burnout. Long, uninteresting training sessions, unrealistic goals, the development of chronic overuse injuries with persistent pain and certain personality types are factors that can predispose towards burnout. The authors believe that it is a crime that young athletes are denied the chance to reach their full human potential because of inappropriate training loads, unrealistic goals and unfeeling coaching techniques. Solutions lie in identifying the problem early, redefining goals and training loads and, if necessary, seeking appropriate professional help from a sports psychologist.

In summary, the long term physical and psychological effects of high level strenuous training on youngsters are not yet fully understood. Regular exercise and physical activity are known to stimulate and enhance normal growth development and health. However, accumulating reports of overuse injury, especially in growing bones, and the effects on growth and maturation of high intensity training indicate a need for concern. Much more research is needed to examine the relationships between injury, the physical and psychological capabilities of young athletes, and the specific skills and training regimes in various sports that are appropriate for children.

PREDISPOSING FACTORS IN THE DEVELOPMENT OF INJURY IN CHILDREN

The developing skeleton has specific growth sites. These growth plates are soft tissue growth cartilage at either end within the shaft of a bone (epiphyses) (fig. 11.1), and at the attachment sites of muscle tendons to the bones (apophyses) (fig. 11.6 and 11.8). These structures allow bone to grow in length and width. Growth plates, being soft tissue structures interposed in hard bone, are consequently sites of weakness that are vulnerable to overuse and traumatic injury.

Growth in humans is not constant; it occurs in spurts. These growth spurts lead to uneven body proportions during the growth period. Consequently, in children there are everchanging leverage and biomechanical forces acting on muscles and joints that are not found in the adult. Therefore, under a given physical loading a child's locomotive apparatus is exposed to greater stress than that of an adult. Hence there is a higher risk of both overuse and traumatic injury, particularly at the most susceptible sites of the growth plates. This risk of injury appears to be particularly acute during rapid growth spurts and recent studies suggest that the peak clinical occurrence is at puberty.

Research has shown that there is a high aerobic cost in children's locomotion. Therefore, for a given exercise load a child will expend much more energy than an adult. The major reason for

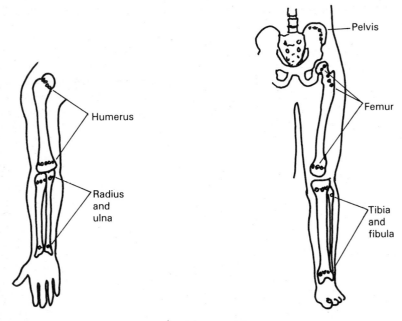

Figure 11.1 Sites of the major limb bones epiphyses.

this appears to be that young children have a more inefficient and wasteful gait resulting in higher energy costs. Therefore, the adult style of training and competition schedules may cause early fatigue and injury in children. Pre-pubescent training should emphasise a good style of locomotion, balance and co-ordination.

Growth spurts also contribute to the onset of injury by increasing the muscle tendon tightness around joints. Growth occurs initially in the long bones and spinal column, therefore increasing the height of the individual. The muscles and tendons increase in length secondary to the skeletal change. Therefore, during growth spurts the bones increase in length first, while the muscles and tendons take time to adapt to the new length, causing a lack of flexibility in the muscles and tendons. Strenuous exercise will enhance this lack of flexibility because of the associated muscle hypertrophy, leaving the muscles, tendons and joint structures vulnerable to injury. However, the major cause for concern are the growth plates which are said to be two to five times weaker than the joint structures and tendons. Therefore, with the inflexibility and tightness of muscles associated with growth spurts and strenuous exercise, this increases the risk of injury at these vulnerable sites.

Recent scientific attention has been given to the correlation between physical performance in sport and the body type of the individual. Studies of international athletes have shown that the best performers in each event or team sport position appear to be drawn from closely matched physical characteristics. Basically, human body types can be divided into three broad categories (fig. 11.2).

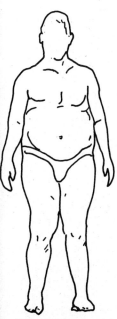 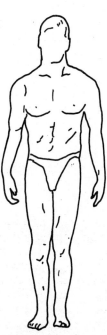 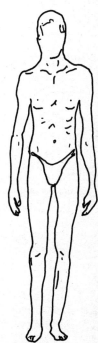

Endomorph

Short and tending to be fat; soft, well rounded body, lacking muscular strength; not adapted to physical activity

Mesomorph

Well muscled, trim, athletic figure, with efficient body movement for physical activity

Ectomorph

Long, lean body, relatively unmuscled; adapted for speed and agility

Figure 11.2   The body types.

Clinical evidence suggests a clear relationship between appropriate body type and injury in sport. For example, the "endomorphic" type child is not suited to contact sports because the greater the amount of soft tissue, the greater the likelihood of soft tissue trauma. These individuals are more suited to sports such as weightlifting, wrestling and long distance swimming. It is reasonable to suggest that top class performance cannot be achieved by the physically unsuitable; the end result is injury. However, this should not preclude a person with an unsuitable body type from participating in a chosen sport, but goals and expectations of performance should be modified accordingly.

A child with a suitable physique and body type for a given sport will not necessarily become a champion. The individual's ability to achieve also depends on his or her psychological makeup, personal goals and environment; the age-old argument of nature versus nurture. Instances of families whose members have made an impact on various sports are legend (the McLean and Ella families in rugby and the Chappells in cricket). It is difficult to determine if these families' sporting prowess is due to genetically inherited or environmental factors, or a combination. Within the Chappell family group, for example, there were strong psychological influences to achieve, opportunites for coaching and experience imparted by family members, in addition to the genetically inherited body type to enable the "elite" performance.

Postural considerations and body alignment factors can also influence the child's ability to perform in selected sports. Poor limb alignment and the associated biomechanical problems in sports such as distance running have been covered extensively in chapter 9, whereas the effects of poor posture, especially on the spine, were discussed in chapter 8. To the authors, the most striking example of the importance of correct posture and body alignment in injury-free performance is in classical dance.

Strain to body structures can easily occur when with incorrect technique poorly aligned limbs are forced into the demands of a sport for which they are not capable. The unusual ballet steps that require dancing on the toes require certain physical attributes. The archetype of a ballet dancer is one with symmetrically balanced upper and lower halves of the body. Pelvis and hips should not be too narrow so as to allow the full 90 degrees turn out of the legs. Lower limb alignment is crucial for excellence in performance.

The legs should be straight with little or no angular deviation. Limb posture that involves malalignments such as bow legs, knocked knees, high riding squinting patellae, rotation of the leg bones and compensatory pronation (the poor alignment syndrome, fig. 9.3) are not suitable for the stress of dance.

Dancers' feet and ankles must have good structure and shape with a formed arch. The arch should not be excessively high (supinated), a position that has poor shock absorption (p.246), or excessively flat (pronated), with its associated problems (p.242). The ideal position the foot should achieve is the neutral position (fig. 9.1). For "pointe" the great, second and third toes should be as close as possible to equal length, as compensatory pronation can cause severe mechanical stress to the feet and legs, especially to the great toe joint leading to the hallux valgus (fig. 9.4 and 9.5).

Every classical dancer must achieve the ultimate range of 90 degrees turnout at the hips. This rotation must be achieved naturally and not by forced muscular effort. The training and stretching to gain this hip rotation must begin at the child's first class. Before the young dancers begin to learn the intricate ballet manoeuvres they must be able to stand without strain in the first three positions of the feet with good hip rotation. Most ballet injuries result from the inability to achieve the full 90 degrees turnout.

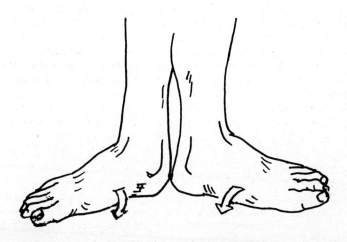

Figure 11.3 ''Rolling in'' — note the collapsed arch of the foot, and the way the first three toes grip the ground.

Dancers who cannot achieve full turnout because of poor technique, forcing inappropriate bodies, or excessively tight hip joint structures, will compensate by adopting two distinctive poor postural positions. First, the dancer will compensate by "rolling in" the forefoot (pronating), gripping the floor with the first three toes and collapsing the arch of the foot (fig. 11.3). This foot posture will cause excessive strain to the great toe joint, the joints of the foot forming the arch, the posterior tibial muscles and the knee and hip joints.

Proper turnout should happen primarily at the hip joint. Dancers who bend their knees forward to achieve a false appearance risk injury. For example, when executing the demi-plié, when incorrect, the knees fall forward of the feet, straining the ligaments of the knees, the patello-femoral joint and also forcing the feet into pronation (rolling in) (fig. 11.4).

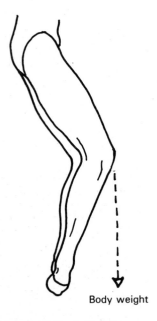 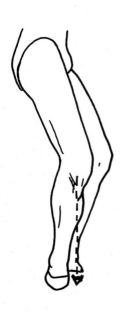

Body weight

a. Incorrect. The knee falls forward, with the weight anterior to the feet, thus stressing the knee joints and flattening the arches of the feet.

b. Correct. Note the weight over the feet and the good alignment of the limbs.

Figure 11.4   Demi-plié; incorrect and correct stances.

In summary we have attempted to show how some people adapt to training better than others, depending on their type of physique, posture and body alignment. When a young athlete is well proportioned and structurally well endowed for the demands of a chosen sport and is under competent guidance, there is little that can go wrong. Most complaints are trivial and a day or two of rest and the appropriate first aid modalities are all that are needed. If pain and symptoms persist for more than a few days, professional advice should be sought.

THE UNIQUE INJURIES OF CHILDREN IN SPORT

EPIPHYSEAL INJURIES

In children, ligaments are three times stronger than the soft cartilage of the growth plate. Therefore, epiphyseal fracture is more likely in children than is damage to the ligaments of a joint.

For example, when a force is applied to the outside of an adult knee a tear of the medial collateral ligament will occur. In the

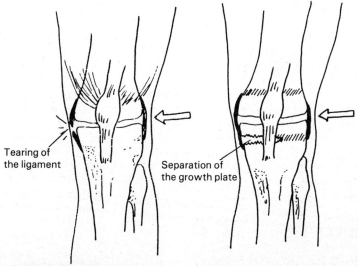

Tearing of
the ligament

Separation of
the growth plate

a. Mechanism of an injury to an adult knee, with a resulting tearing of the medial ligament.

b. Mechanism of an injury to a child's knee, with a resulting injury to the growth plate.

Figure 11.5   Comparison of an adult's knee injury with that of a child.

knee of a child the medial collateral ligament inserts into the soft epiphyses of the tibia and femur. When force is applied to the outside of the child's knee there is more likelihood of epiphyseal fracture than of ligament damage (fig. 11.5).

When a child presents with evidence of a dislocation, fracture or sprain, an epiphyseal fracture should be suspected. A thorough medical examination and, where necessary, the appropriate X-rays, should be undertaken. Any diagnosis of a severe sprain that does not improve after an appropriate period of time and treatment should be re-examined for an undisplaced or unrecognised epiphyseal fracture.

In general, undisplaced epiphyseal fractures are successfully treated by immobilisation for two to four weeks and then the patient is given a rehabilitation program to return to full strength, power, endurance and flexibility. With a displaced fracture, surgical procedures are often needed to align the fragments properly.

Most epiphyseal injuries heal satisfactorily. However, there are some complications that can occur. Because the epiphyses are growing areas they have a vibrant blood supply. Fracture of the epiphyseal growth plate may disrupt blood vessels and lead to the death of bone, producing bony fragments (osteochondritis dissecans). In severe fractures, disturbances of bone growth may occur and such disturbances may not be identified for months after injury to a growth plate.

The epiphyses are also susceptible to overuse injury as well as direct trauma. The most susceptible are the growth centres of the long bones of the lower limbs and feet. As stated previously, little research has been done on the long term effects of too stressful training loads on growing bones. Recent studies have shown that excessive pressure placed on growth plates, such as rapid increases in running distances and the frequency of exercise, can lead to stress fractures of the epiphyses. Other studies suggest that prolonged, excessive loading of the epiphyses will cause their premature closure, hence a reduction in the stature of the child.

APOPHYSEAL INJURIES

These injuries are "traction" injuries to the growth plates that are associated with the insertions of the major muscle tendons to the bone (apophysis). Injury can occur to any apophyseal site; however, the authors have selected the major sites of injury for discussion.

Osgood Schlatter's Disease

This condition is one of the most common sources of knee pain that the authors see in the young pre-adolescent athletes.

Anatomy

The large patella tendon, which is the tendon of insertion of all the powerful quadriceps muscles, attaches to the tibia. To allow this bony attachment to grow in width, height and strength, there is an apophysis situated between it and the tibia (fig. 11.6).

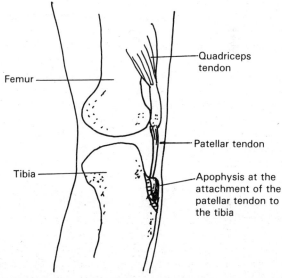

Figure 11.6 The soft growth plate (apophysis) at the attachment of the patellar tendon to the tibia.

Excessive traction placed on this growth plate leads to pain, inflammation and swelling of the front upper part of the lower leg.

Causes of Injury

The major factor in the development of Osgood Schlatter's disease is a fault of training. The various training faults are discussed in full in chapter 9. Mistakes in training loads will place excessive tractional stress on the growth plate (apophysis) causing breakdown of the soft tissue structure leading to inflammation, swelling, pain and a decrease in the ability to perform.

Children are more susceptible to overuse injury during times of growth spurts. As discussed previously, bony growth takes place before muscle length can accommodate the increase in length. When coupled with muscle hypertrophy and a decrease in flexibility due to training, a situation develops where excessive traction is placed on the apophysis and injury occurs. In Osgood Schlatter's disease the quadriceps and hamstring muscles become inflexible, causing increased force to be applied across the knee extensor mechanism and the growth plate.

Adolescents with the "poor limb alignment" syndrome (fig. 9.3) are particularly susceptible to this injury. The anatomical malalignment and the tortional effects placed on the limb with "overpronation" can multiply the stresses placed on the growth plate. The mechanism of injury is the same as described in the role of limb alignment and compensatory pronation in the development of peripatellar stress syndrome (runner's knee), on page 270, chapter 9. It is quite common for young athletes presenting with Osgood Schlatter's to also suffer from symptoms arising from peripatellar stress and tendonitis of the patellar tendon (jumper's knee, page 273).

Signs and Symptoms

There is usually no history of injury except a progressive increase in pain with activity. In the early stages the pain is relieved with rest from sport, only to return as sport is resumed. In advanced cases, the inflammatory process can be so severe that there is a constant ache which is made worse with physical activity.

Most patients will present with a bulbous hard "lump" on the front of the knee (fig. 11.7). This lump is quite tender to palpation. X-rays may show a widening of the gap between the bony muscle

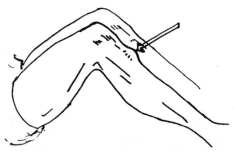

Figure 11.7 The bulbous lump on the front of the knee, characteristic of Osgood-Schlatter's disease.

insertion and the shaft of the tibia denoting a traction injury to the growth plate. The pain is usually made worse with active straightening of the knee, especially against resistance. The symptoms often occur in both knees.

Sever's Disease

This variety of heel pain is often confused with Achilles tendonitis. The injury is a traction injury to the apophysis where the large Achilles tendon inserts onto the heel bone (calcaneum) (fig. 11.8).

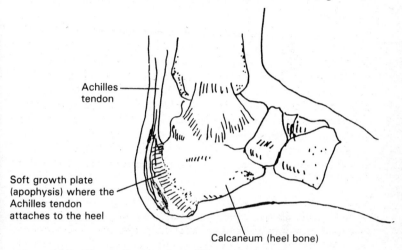

Achilles tendon

Soft growth plate (apophysis) where the Achilles tendon attaches to the heel

Calcaneum (heel bone)

Figure 11.8   The apophysis at the Achilles tendon insertion.

Signs and Symptoms

This condition is usually seen in children in the age range of about 8 to 13 years. They present with painful, tender heels. The pain is made worse with sport and activity and relieved with rest, except in the chronic cases. Often this injury is associated with Achilles tendonitis.

Cause of Injury

Similar factors to those that contribute to Achilles tendonitis apply to the development of Sever's disease. The growth plate, being weaker than the tendon, is the site of injury in children as opposed to the tendon in adults. The overuse factors involved in the development of injury to the Achilles insertion complex include:

training faults, anatomical factors such as malalignment and overpronation, and environmental factors such as inappropriate shoes and shoe wear. All these factors are covered in depth throughout this book, especially in chapter 6 in the section dealing with "Achilles tendonitis" (p.258).

In the authors' experience, the chief cause of injury is a combination of the factors just outlined, coupled with the problems associated with rapid growth. The calf muscles of young athletes hypertrophy with training and competition. During growth spurts the bones increase in length at the expense of muscle flexibility, therefore developing very tight calf muscles and Achilles tendon. This situation is common in all athletes but particularly so in highland dancing where the type of dance step does not permit the heel to lower. This accentuates the development of tight calf muscle-tendon units. This excessive calf muscle tightness, particularly when associated with malalignment and compensatory pronation, will cause strong traction forces to be applied to the apophyseal plate at the heel leading to pain, inflammation and swelling.

Other Common Sites of Apophyseal Injury

Traction apophysitis can occur at the insertion of any major muscle involved in sports action. At the elbow, apophyseal injury to the common forearm flexor muscles attachment to the medial epicondyle (fig. 10.10) can occur in throwing sports, especially baseball pitching and javelin throwing. The mechanism of injury is the same as described in "thrower's elbow" (chapter 10). In children, however, the apophyseal plate is weaker than the medial collateral ligament of the elbow so the damage occurs at the soft growth plate instead of the adult ligamentous injury.

In the pelvic and hip regions there are attachments of major muscle groups that are involved in running. These sites of muscle insertion are consequently sites of apophyseal injury in the growing child. (Fig. 11.9 illustrates the most common areas where injury can occur.)

The Treatment of Apophyseal Injury

These injuries are an overstressing of the soft tissue growth plates; therefore they have the signs and symptoms common to all soft tissue injury, that is, pain, inflammation, swelling and local tenderness. Thus, treatment follows the principles applied throughout this book to the management of soft tissue injury.

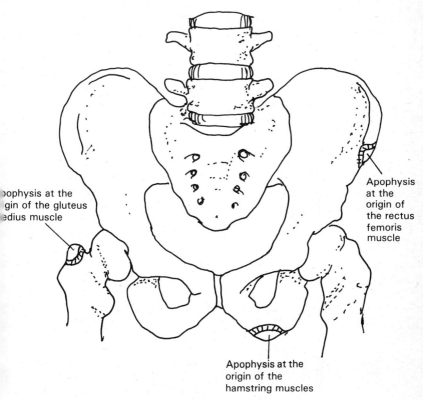

Apophysis at the origin of the gluteus medius muscle

Apophysis at the origin of the rectus femoris muscle

Apophysis at the origin of the hamstring muscles

Figure 11.9   Common pelvic muscle insertion sites of apophyseal injuries.

The first aid modality of choice is naturally I.C.E. applied using the techniques described in chapter 3. In the initial stages rest from pain is the most important modality of treatment. Any activity that causes further pain and swelling is only increasing the damage to the growth plate. Chronically severe and painful cases may even require a short period of immobilisation. This is an extreme measure only to be used when all else fails because of the muscle wastage and stiffening of joint structures inherent in any prolonged immobilisation.

Physiotherapy modalities can quickly reduce the pain and inflammation and are a valuable tool in providing symptomatic relief for children's injuries without having to resort to drugs. The major role of the sports physiotherapist is to assess and correct the factors responsible for the development of the injury. Rest alone will not resolve the problem. Complete pain-free return to activity requires the correction of underlying fault(s). Thus the sports physiotherapist, to manage the injury comprehensively, will:

1 correct the underlying training error and supervise the young athlete's progressive return to sport;

2 apply the correct stretching techniques to counter "muscle inflexibility": for example, (a) in Osgood Schlatter's disease, the stretches for the quadriceps and hamstrings (fig. 1.3(b) and 1.3(d)); (b) Sever's disease, stretches to the calf complex (fig. 1.3(g));

3 assess alignment and postural anomalies and prescribe the appropriate corrective exercise and/or recommend podiatry management;

4 prescribe a comprehensive rehabilitation program to ensure a complete return to full strength, power, endurance and flexibility to the damaged area. For example, in a longstanding case of Osgood Schlatter's disease, wastage of the quadriceps muscles will occur, particularly the vastus medialis oblique (VMO). The VMO's action is to stabilise the patella (fig. 9.26) and if the wastage is not corrected the knee then becomes susceptible to the added problem of peripatellar pain.

THE PREVENTION OF CHILDREN'S INJURY IN SPORT

Young children are not miniature adults, they are growing organisms in the process of physical and mental maturation. Consequently, training programs, competitive playing schedules and rules applied to many sports and games are not always appropriate for the growing child. Sport has beneficial effects on health, fitness, and physiological function, and life-long value as recreation and relaxation. These positive aspects should be emphasised by physical educators, coaches and parents in devising sporting programs for young children. The adult goals of "fierce competition" and "winning at all costs" are not appropriate for growing bodies.

There are no concrete answers to the questions surrounding training, competition and their association with the development of injury in children. However, there are certain guidelines that can help parents and coaches to make decisions on the training loads that they give their children.

- Treat young athletes as children first and athletes second. Children are not mentally or physically capable of the same exertion and effort as adult athletes. Children usually do not drive themselves to the point of injury unless unreasonable demands are placed on them by coaches and parents.
- Competition and training demands that are appropriate for adults are not appropriate for children who are physically and psychologically not mature enough to withstand such pressure. For 5-to-10-year-olds emphasis should be placed on fun, awakening interest in sport and health and developing basic skills, especially in balance and co-ordination. For 10-to-15-year-olds emphasis should be placed on the acquisition of the skills and techniques of sport and developing a tolerance for increased training loads. The 15-to-18-year-olds are ready to be exposed to heavier training loads and be involved in weight training and high levels of competition.
- Grouping of children for sport should take into consideration factors such as size, weight, physical maturation, physical condition and skill level. Age is not an appropriate criterion because there are a wide range of developmental levels in any growing age group. There should be no reason to separate pre-adolescent children by sex in sport or recreation. However, the authors feel that females should not participate against pubescent and post-pubescent males in contact or collision sports.
- Specialisation in a particular sport is not appropriate until after puberty. Because of the hormonal changes and other factors associated with puberty, a child who shows potential in a given sport pre-puberty might then develop other characteristics that are not advantageous to his chosen sport after puberty. In the young athlete emphasis should be given to the introduction to as many sports as possible and specialisation should not occur until the child is 10 to 12 years old.
- Children should be supervised in organised sport and recreation by competent officials. There is a need for greater emphasis, in the education and accreditation of coaches and educators, on the special needs of our younger athletes.
- Rules of the games that are appropriate for adults should be modified for young children. Game, practice and season length must also be appropriate for the developmental level of the athletes. The increased emphasis on specialisation in

one sport has lead to the situation where children as young as seven and eight years are training and competing ten to eleven months a year. Young children should be restricted to seasons of no longer than six to eight weeks with two to three practice sessions and one competition game per week.

- The concepts of injury prevention discussed in chapter 1 are just as applicable to children as they are to adults. The factors that are particularly essential for children are *flexibility* and the *warm-up/down*. As discussed constantly throughout this section, muscle inflexibility, associated with hypertrophy and growth spurts, is one of the major precursors of injury in children.

READING LIST

INJURIES AND MANAGEMENT

PRIMARY READING

Australian Sports Medicine Federation. 1986.
The sports trainer. Care and prevention of sporting injuries.
Sydney: Jacaranda Press.
Beiersdorf, 1979.
Modern sports strapping and bandaging techniques.
Sydney: Beiersdorf (Aust.) Ltd
Dornan, P. 1980.
Sporting injuries: A trainer's guide.
Brisbane: University of Queensland Press.
Gibbs, R. 1982.
Sporting injuries: Prevention, first aid and after care.
2nd ed. Melbourne: Sun Books
Hood, M. 1980.
Preparation, performance and patch-up: A guide to fitness training and injury prevention.
Auckland: Heinemann Publishers.
Mirkin, G. and Hoffman, M. 1978.
The sports medicine book.
Boston: Little Brown & Co.
Muckle, D.S. 1980.
Injuries in sport.
Bristol: John Wright & Sons.
St Johns Ambulance. 1980.
First aid.
2nd ed. Melbourne
Stokes, P.G. 1979.
A guide to sports medicine.
Philadelphia: Saunders.

ADVANCED READING

Allman, F.L. and Ryan, A.J. 1974.
Sports medicine.
New York: Academic Press.

Klafs, C.E. and Arnheim, D.D. 1985.
Modern principles of athletic training.
6th ed. St Louis: C.V. Mosby.

Peterson, L. and Renstrom, P. 1986.
Sports injuries: Their prevention and treatment.
Sydney: Methuen (Aust.) Pty Ltd.

Roy, S. and Irvin, R. 1983.
Sports medicine: Prevention, evaluation, management and rehabilitation.
Englewood Cliffs, N.J.: Prentice Hall.

Williams, J.G.P. 1980.
A colour atlas of injury in sport.
Wolfe Medical Publications.

Williams, J.G.P. 1980.
Injury in sport.
Wolfe Medical Publications.

OTHER SPORTS MEDICINE TOPICS

Astrand, P. and Rodahl, K. 1977.
Textbook of work physiology.
New York:McGraw-Hill.

Donald, K. 1983.
The doping game.
Brisbane: Boolarong Publications.

Inge, K. and Brukner, P. 1986.
Food for sport.
Melbourne: W. Heinemann.

INDEX